Washing Ourselves Sick

S. B. McEwen

Table of Contents

Jenny is a fictional character. Her actions are real; her crises are real. We all have a little Jenny in each of us.

Dedication

To my dad, I wish you were here to see this book.

Author's Note

I have a background in germs. Specifically, I have an undergraduate degree in molecular biology/ biotechnology and a master's degree in microbiology. I have spent a lot of time studying germs, bacteria, and viruses and learning about the immune system. I have had a lot of experience with germs both in instructional laboratories and employment. Personally, I have always had a belief that exposure to germs, bacteria, and viruses was not a terrible thing to the healthy individual. The more exposure one has to germs, the better the natural ability to fight off infections using your own immune system, like immune system exercise. After all, that is why you have an immune system.

Besides education, I often think back to childhood. I did not grow up unclean, far from it as I was not allowed to walk on the vacuum marks my mom put in the carpet, but I did grow up doing things like swimming in the Allegheny River and playing in an old sandbox or on a rusty swing set. I ate the loaf of bread that had one moldy slice because the other slices were still good. Things many people today may find "dirty." Maybe my view on germs is a little old-fashioned. My kids were thumb-suckers, thus they touched everything, then put their thumbs in their mouths. Yes, I found it a little disgusting at times, but they were not any more sick than other kids I knew, so I chalked it up to building immunity. I emphasized handwashing with soap and water, trying my hardest not to use, or let others use on my kids, things like the chemical-laden, alcohol-based hand sanitizers. I am honestly afraid of this "overclean" world. I am afraid that we are doing more harm than good.

Today, society is creating a worldwide fear about contagious disease and the cleaning and sanitizing of everything. Hand sanitizers and disinfectant cleaners are given special priority in store displays. Hand-sanitizing dispensers and sanitizing stations with wipes and cleaners are everywhere—grocery stores, offices, churches, and schools just to name a few. People are becoming extreme germophobes with a "germ-free" environment as the ultimate goal.

This overclean fear has been on my mind for years, but when the COVID pandemic hit, I could not keep my thoughts to myself. Everyone racing to buy cleaning and sanitizing agents to rid themselves of any and all germs was the final straw for me. All the arguments and ideas I had on natural immunity and putting that immunity to use became the words on these pages. Through research on my thoughts, I also learned a lot that solidified my opinions. There is a list of references in the back of this book. I invite you to utilize the list should you like to read more on any of the topics.

This book is not about COVID or pandemics or any other bacterial or viral outbreak. I mention COVID or data from the year 2020 several times as this pandemic and the response by society is relatable and the data is recent. However, most of the incidents discussed in this book are events of pre-COVID or non-pandemic times.

I hope you enjoy the book. My goal is to raise awareness of the dangers of an overclean mentality and the potential harm we are doing to ourselves and our families. I will let you decide for yourself if you think we are cleaning ourselves to a healthier life or *Washing Ourselves Sick.*

Hmm . . . Really?

In 2020, poison control centers documented 24,802 cases of exposure poisoning from hand sanitizer in children. Exposure poisoning being contact, or exposure, to a toxin or poison. These incidences can be anything from skin contact to ingestion, accidental or intentional. And these 24,802 cases are just in the age group 0–12 years old.

As time progresses, society is focusing more and more on sanitizing every surface of everything. New products are continuously being released to clean and sanitize things we never thought to be laden with bacteria or viruses. What is not publicized or advertised are the studies being released showing that use of household cleaning products is being linked to lung cancer, breast cancer, and even infertility and possibly autoimmune disease.

Now think of your day. How often do you rub hand sanitizer on your hands? Do you know how long it takes for the sanitizer to be in contact with the bacteria to actually be effective? How about children using hand sanitizers, maybe your children or children you know or see in public? Do you see small children being given a squirt after playing on a playground or before having a snack? Most likely that answer is yes. Some hand sanitizers have twice as much alcohol per volume as vodka. Do you see parents squirting vodka on their kids' hands? Most likely that answer is no.

How about cleaning and disinfecting other solid surfaces? How often do you wipe down your countertops in your kitchen? What do you wipe your counters with? Do you even think to rinse the chemical cleaners off your counters before placing food on the surface? How often do you clean other surfaces like railings, toilet seats, and light switches? Do you spray Lysol on your shoes when you enter your house? How about outside your home? Do you disinfect the grocery cart handle or your car's steering wheel?

In this book, you will meet Jenny, a young mom trying to do the best she can to love, care for, and keep her children safe. We follow her through her habits of cleaning and disinfecting. You may relate to Jenny's habits, or you may find her extreme. You may realize you are just like Jenny, or maybe only like her in a few ways. You will read about what Jenny does on a regular basis and how she is helping or harming herself and her family, sometimes both. Also, you will learn some of the frightening events that could happen from hand sanitizer and excessive cleaning product usage. Although Jenny is a fictional character, all the events happening to her on these pages are real events.

You will learn the risks to your own health due to the combination of sanitizers on your skin and disinfectants on household and daily objects. With hand sanitizer, you are destroying the tiny ecosystems existing on your own hands that help you defend yourself against disease while leaving behind physical dirt. You are exposing yourself to toxins and carcinogens in cleaning products. You may even be weakening your immune system, setting yourself up for autoimmune disease. So now ask yourself this question: Are you cleaning your life of harmful bacteria and viruses, or are you washing yourself sick?

Washing Ourselves Sick

This Is My Friend Jenny

Meet Jenny.

Jenny is a mother in her mid-30s. She grew up in middle-class suburbia of western Pennsylvania, in a little town where she walked to school. As a school-child, Jenny made good grades and kept herself out of trouble. Although not extraordinarily popular, Jenny had a lot of friends.

Jenny went on to a larger university in Virginia to study business, majoring in marketing. At college, she met her husband, Jake, an accountant. Married for nine years, they now live together in a nice family-oriented neighbor-hood not far from where Jenny grew up in western Pennsylvania. After just a few years of wedded bliss—the double-income-no-kids kind of life—Jenny put her career on hold to start a family.

Now Jenny is the very blessed mother of three children. Her oldest, Brock, is a brown-haired 7-year-old boy in second grade. As most boys are, he is very active, has playdates with classmates after school, and is also involved in soccer and flag football. The middle child is a 4-year-old curly-haired girl, Veronica, Ronnie for short. She attends preschool three half days a week. Ronnie also has playdates, usually after the half day at school. Weather permitting in western PA, Ronnie loves to go to the park to look for pretty flowers and leaves or to the playground to swing. Jenny's third child is a little 18-month-old daughter, Harper, who has sprouts of fine blond hair. The little one is in playgroups with friends, maybe more like a playgroup with Jenny's friends, but a regular time for age-appropriate socialization for both mom and daughter. Jenny is a great mother, very attentive to her children, and she is sure to keep all of her children occupied socially and physically. She wants her children to be raised in a loving environment where they not only learn academically but also learn about taking care of themselves and others. She wants her kids to be healthy, both disease-free and lifestyle active.

Jenny still keeps her foot in the door of a career by doing a little consulting work on the side, but her real job is the health and well-being of her family. She prides herself in keeping a clean home, a little cluttered at times with three kids but germ-free clean. In the little free time she has, like nap time and later in the evenings after the kids have gone to bed, Jenny reads. She enjoys reading parenting magazines and books and, of course, browsing social media. Social media keeps Jenny up to date on the latest "bug" going around her local school. She is very attentive to this information as she does not want her children to be the start of a school-wide stomach flu or the heated topic on the schools "Moms of Elementary School" page. In her reading and browsing, she is told to keep her kids from others who are sick, keep her children from those who are not vaccinated, and keep her kids and home germ-free. Advertisements are everywhere for antibacterials and sanitizers. She takes to this information like the Bible. After all, she wants to raise healthy, happy children.

Information about cleanliness and germ-free lifestyles is everywhere. Jenny sees commercials during her morning talk shows, which, of course, she has on as background because she is way too busy to sit and watch TV. These commercials push for products that sanitize your laundry, your sofa, and there's even a tiny box that can sterilize your cell phone. When doing errands, Jenny sees dispensers for hand sanitizer in store entryways and disinfectant wipes for grocery carts. Even when shopping for a new dishwasher, she is sold on the model with the "sanitizing cycle." Surely her kids are not going to eat off germ-ridden plates!

The following pages are stories about Jenny. Mostly the everyday habits Jenny has adopted for cleaning and disinfecting. For example, Jenny loves to use hand sanitizer as she is concerned about what she or her children touch and the germs they acquire. Also, she cleans and disinfects her entire home, countertops, laundry, stuffed animals, etc. Follow Jenny through some of her everyday habits. Note the crises Jenny experiences, some of which Jenny brings on herself, all with the best of intentions for health and wellness for her family. Is there such a thing as too much disinfecting and sanitizing? Is Jenny being healthy, or is she washing herself sick?

Washing Ourselves Sick

Grapes of Wrath

One spring day, Jenny was meeting her sister at McDonald's for lunch. Ronnie went home with a friend after preschool, and Brock was in school all day, so she was taking Harper, her little 18-month-old daughter. To add some healthy options to the chicken nuggets, Jenny packed grapes and cheese cubes. Jenny found a small booth table and a high chair. After setting her purse and diaper bag on the table, she removed a sanitizing wipe from her purse and wiped down the high chair before she securely buckled her toddler into the seat. She then moved her purse and diaper bag to the booth seat. Jenny opened her purse, removed a bottle of hand sanitizer, and squirted the table. Using a restaurant napkin, she wiped off the sanitizer. Next Jenny opened the diaper bag and removed the grapes and cheese, which were cut up into smaller than bite-size pieces, and set them on the bare table. After all, Jenny thought the table was now clean and sterile.

Now let's think about what was really on that fast-food table, or maybe you would rather not think about it, but we are going to anyway. The prior customer had his elbows on the table, his hands on the table, and he placed the napkin he used to wipe his mouth on the table. That prior customer had a teenage son that used the bathroom, did not wash his hands, and returned to the table to sit with his hands and elbows across the table. But Jenny cleaned the table with hand sanitizer, right?

Just how effective are hand sanitizers? Let's look. Hand-sanitizing products containing 90% alcohol advertise killing 99.9% of bacteria and viruses. That sounds pretty effective, but to achieve this 99.9% effective rate, the sanitizer needs to be in contact with bacteria and viruses for at least 30 seconds. Sure, killing 99.9% of bacteria sounds great, but that still leaves 0.1% of bacteria remaining, assuming 30 seconds of contact. What does 0.1% represent? As an easy example, consider bacteria and a common surface like the handle of a kitchen faucet. The number of bacteria is measured in colony-forming units or CFUs. Colony-forming units are defined as bacteria that have the ability to multiply and grow, often a cluster of bacteria, not just one individual microscopic bacterium. When counting in CFUs, dead bacteria are not counted. There are approximately 228,854 bacterial colony units on the average handle of a kitchen faucet . . . per square inch. If we keep only 0.1% of those bacterial colonies, we still have 229 colonies remaining per square inch. In other words, bacteria that are living can still be alive after being in contact with the directed 30 seconds of hand sanitizer. And remember, this is a handle of a kitchen faucet and Jenny was at a fast-food restaurant.

Table 1 shows common surfaces and the number of bacteria units, CFUs, present on those surfaces as well as the number of living bacteria remaining after contact with 90% alcohol sanitizer. The data in table 1 also assumes 30-second contact between bacteria and sanitizer. In looking at table 1, there are still many viable, live bacteria left after a 30-second exposure to 90% alcohol sanitizer. The common range of alcohol in sanitizers is 65–95%. Therefore, some sanitizers will leave more bacterial colony-forming units than listed in table 1.

Bacterial Colony-Forming Units per Square Inch on Common Items

Surface	CFUs untreated	CFUs remaining after 30-second exposure to 90% alcohol-based hand sanitizer
Dish Sponge	775,460,560	775,461
Kitchen Faucet Handle	228,854	229
Shopping Cart	138,000	138
Computer Mouse	79,000	79
Toilet Seat	1,201	1
Cutting Board	61,597	62
Kitchen Countertop	1,736	2
Self-Checkout Screen	4,500	5
Doorknob	8,643	9
Cell Phone	11,020	11
Remote Control	17,000	17
Bathroom Faucet	50,068	50

Table 1. Number of colony-forming units (CFUs) present on average daily items. A CFU is a living bacterial cluster large

enough to form a visible colony. Dead colonies are not counted. Note the toilet seat versus the cell phone.

Thinking about Jenny's table, maybe the table was cleaned by employees between customers. Maybe the table was washed with a clean cloth and solution of disinfectant and left to air-dry, thus exposing the table to the disinfectant for a good 30–60 seconds. Remember when Jenny came to the table? She placed her purse and diaper bag on the table while strapping her toddler into the highchair. Where else has her purse been? Most likely, Jenny's purse had been on her car floor, the same car floor where shoes worn in a public bathroom have touched. Her purse was in a grocery cart where hundreds of hands and maybe raw chicken have been. Jenny's purse was hanging on the back of the public bathroom door. Many studies have concluded that purse bottoms and purse handles are some of the dirtiest places around. Quite often even things like *E. coli* are found on purse bottoms.

There were probably germs, bacteria, and viruses already on the surface of the table. However, if they were not already there, they were deposited there by the things we put on the table, like the purse. I am sure you are saying, "But Jenny wiped the table with hand sanitizer, so it must be clean." Jenny squirted and wiped in about 5 seconds to clean her table. There was no 30-second exposure to the germs. After all, she was juggling a toddler at the same time as sanitizing. There is a minimum of 0.1% of bacteria (fungi and viruses too) remaining on the table. Would you spread your toddler's lunch on that table?

Would You Rub Alcohol on Your Heart?

Jenny, unbeknownst to herself, is classified as a germaphobe. A germaphobe is defined as someone obsessed with cleanliness and terrified of germs. She even falls under the diagnosis of mysophobia, a condition of compulsive hand cleaning to avoid all types of germs.

> Mysophobia, also known as verminophobia, germophobia, germaphobia, bacillophobia, and bacteriophobia, is a pathological fear of contamination and germs. The term was coined by William A. Hammond in 1879 when describing a case of obsessive-compulsive disorder exhibited in repeatedly washing one's hands. Mysophobia has long been related to compulsive hand washing. Names pertaining directly to the abnormal fear of dirt and filth include molysmophobia or molysomophobia, rhypophobia, and rupophobia, whereas the terms bacillophobia and bacteriophobia specifically refer to the fear of bacteria and microbes in general. (Wikipedia)

One habit Jenny had was her use of hand sanitizer on her hands. She kept a bottle in her car, a bottle attached to her purse strap, a dispenser in her kitchen, and another bottle by her toddlers' changing area. She used hand sanitizer often throughout the day. She took a squirt and rubbed it into her hands until it dried any time she entered the grocery store, left the grocery store, went to the park with her toddler, entered church, left church, returned home from anywhere, before cooking dinner, after checking her mail from her mailbox, etc. etc. etc. Because of this frequent use, Jenny's hands were dry and cracked.

Hand sanitizers contain a large amount of alcohol. Up to 95% of hand sanitizer can be alcohol. Alcohol is a necessary component of hand sanitizer as it is the ingredient that kills the germs. (Bacteria actually pop, destroying their protective cell wall, in the presence of alcohol much like a bubble-gum bubble pops when overinflated.) Alcohol is used in sanitizing products because of its ability to be a broad-spectrum sanitizing agent. Broad spectrum in reference to alcohol means alcohol can kill a wide range, broad spectrum of bacteria. Also, alcohol does not diminish the effectiveness of other agents such as degreasers or moisturizers that may be added ingredients.

Using hand sanitizer and its effects on our skin is a catch-22. The higher the alcohol content of the sanitizer, the more germs are killed. However, the higher the alcohol content of the sanitizer, the more detrimental to our skin. Many people using sanitizers regularly experience very dry, cracked, irritated skin.

This dryness can lead to aging of the skin on the hands. Since hands can tell a person's age, premature aging of the hands is not a desirable effect. Frequent users of hand sanitizer often suffer from contact dermatitis, itchy, red, and irritated skin. Why does this matter? Because your umbrella has holes!

Dry, cracked hands to your immune system is like using an umbrella with holes.

Here is a trivia question. What is your largest organ? Answer: Your skin! Yes, your skin is an organ. Your skin encloses your bones, muscles, circulatory system, and internal organs. Your skin also serves as insulation for your body and keeps you from losing excessive water. Skin, also, is the first line of defense in keeping germs from entering the body. Cracked skin means germs can get through our skin barrier and into our deep tissues and circulatory system. In context to excessive sanitizing, dry, cracked hands to your immune system is like using an umbrella with holes.

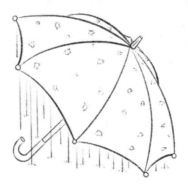

Skin, in a natural, unsanitized state, has resident bacteria. Bacteria start colonizing your body the moment you are born. You cannot get rid of them, no matter how many times a day you take a shower or wash. On your skin, there are an average of 32 million bacteria for every 1 square inch of your skin. However, do not let that number stress you out—all of those billions of skin bacteria combined would fit into a ball the size of a pea.

It is very important to remember that most of the bacteria that live on your skin are either no threat to you, the host, or beneficial! Yes, beneficial to the host, which means beneficial to you! The beneficial bacteria can perform two different functions. One role beneficial bacteria can take is releasing substances that prevent harmful bacteria from living (colonizing) on your skin. Think of this like spraying cooking spray on your skillet when you hear an egg is about to be cooked. These bacteria release substances that prevent harmful bacteria from sticking around. For example, *Corynebacterium accolens* is a natural inhabitant of the skin. It releases an antibacterial to inhibit the growth of another bacteria, *Streptococcus pneumoniae*. The latter bacteria being the causative agent of pneumonia.

The second role of beneficial bacteria is they can produce the warning signal to the immune system to induce an immune response. Think of these bacteria like an alarm system in your home. When the alarm goes off, you are alerted that your safety zone has been compromised and you need to take action. Defend yourself or call the police. These skin bacteria can send a signal to your immune system, starting a reaction to send immune cells to defend themselves against the intruding germ. This second role of beneficial bacteria can be explained with the skin inhabitant *Staphylococcus epidermidis*. These bacteria are one of the most common inhabitants of the skin, and when triggered, they can start the body to mount an immune response against other bacterial infections or fungi.

Local Community Facebook Survey

Behavior of Hand Sanitizer Use	Percentage Exhibiting Behavior
Occasional use, especially when out in public a lot	40.5
Many times throughout the day	20.5
Only when access to soap and water are not available	28.5
Only when asked by an establishment, store, or school	7.5
Never	3

Table 2. Facebook survey. Random survey asking how often people use hand sanitizers. (McEwen)

A recent public Facebook survey was posted asking random people, not just friends, what their hand-sanitizing habits are. (Table 2) The survey was essentially asking if people use hand sanitizer and how often. The results show that Jenny's behavior is not uncommon.

Surveying a local community, people were asked how often they used sanitizer given the following choices for answers:

- Occasionally, especially when out in public a lot
- Only when access to soap/water is not available
- Many times throughout the day
- Only when asked by an establishment, store, or school
- Never

Over half the people answered they use sanitizer regularly throughout the day and/or when they are out in public a lot. About 29% answered they only use hand sanitizers when they do not have access to soap and water. Fewer than 8% polled said they only use sanitizers when requested by a store, establishment, or school. The smallest category was 3% answering "never." Given this data, about 3% of people are keeping their skin completely intact as their first line of defense, and about 36% are keeping their immune umbrella from getting holes on a regular basis.

In other words, over half the people taking the survey may have an umbrella with holes out in the rain.

If your skin is dry and cracked, your defensive line is cracked. Although the sanitizing kills germs, those few remaining germs as well as newly contacted germs now have an easier time entering our bodies through dry, cracked skin.

So many people are willing to rub alcohol over their hands multiple times a day, in fear of germs, not realizing the damaging effects to their skin and possibly their overall immune health. Would you rub alcohol over your heart several times a day? Of course not, because the heart is an important organ. Your skin, including the skin on your hands, is also an important organ. So why rub alcohol-based sanitizers on your hands?

On another note, and in Jenny's defense, remember that not all bacteria on your skin are helpful. Yes, the germophobes and Jennys out there will be happy to hear that some bacteria on your skin can harm you or make you sick. Technically, these bacteria are called pathogens. Go back to the concept about hand sanitizer drying your skin and causing cracks in your hands. Remember the umbrella with holes analogy? There are pathogenic bacteria on your skin naturally that will be able to penetrate your organ barrier, aka skin, when your hands get dry and cracked.

Now put the concepts of beneficial bacteria residing on our hands with the fact that pathogenic bacteria reside on our hands in combination with what is being done with usage of hand sanitizers. Overuse of drying agents like alcohol-rich sanitizers cause cracks in your skin barrier. We have our own little community of bacteria naturally living on our skin, specifically our hands. Left alone to normal handwashing with soap and water, dirt and bacteria are washed away but not entirely stripped. The skin, our important organ of self-defense, is left intact. Put down the hand sanitizer and keep your umbrella from getting holes.

The Dirty Diaper

Once a week on Jenny's calendar was playgroup for Harper, her 18-month-old toddler. Last week, Jenny was the playgroup host. Four moms, three of Jenny's friends plus Jenny, got together with their little ones ranging in age from 11 months to age 2. Playgroup was a time where both the little ones and the moms got some quality socialization. Jenny looked forward to these playdates. She got a chance to catch up with her friends on the latest trends, recipes, and let us be honest, gossip. Usually when they all got together, the little ones played while the moms talked. Everyone had a light lunch, and the kids returned to playtime until someone had a meltdown indicating the playdate had ended.

At this last playgroup Jenny hosted at her home, Harper had a dirty diaper. Harper's timing was impeccable because Jenny was just beginning to prep lunch—salad for the ladies and cut-up fruit and mac-and-cheese for the little ones. The kids were getting cranky, and Jenny was trying to prep quickly when she realized the dirty diaper smell in the room was coming from her child. So she snatched her little one up and carried her to the changing table. Quickly, Jenny got the fresh diaper and lavender-scented baby wipes ready. Jenny had done this hundreds of times, so she was on autopilot. She removed the soiled diaper, wiped the toddler's bottom clean, and put on the clean fresh diaper. Jenny rolled up all the smelly garbage and placed it in a bag. Next to the changing table of her toddler was, as you would expect from Jenny, a bottle of hand sanitizer. After disposing of the stinky diaper, Jenny squirted her hand sanitizer into her hands, rubbed her hands, and waved them in the air until dry. She picked up Harper quickly to go back to her friends and the playgroup. After all, the kids were hungry, and she was in a hurry to get back to preparing lunch. Hand sanitizer was quicker and far more convenient than washing with soap and water.

Most germ-fearing people mistake sanitized for clean.

Yes, Jenny changed a dirty diaper with her bare hands, then sanitized before going back to her playgroup. Jenny's hands were clean, right? Now she could go back to preparing her salad, mac-and-cheese, and cut fruit. Jenny's hands might have been sterile, but not necessarily clean. In the definition of the word clean, there is no reference or synonym to the word sterile. Jenny's hands might have been sterile, but there was a good possibility that she had a little fecal matter on her hands from the diaper change, just now it was sterile fecal matter. And the fecal matter being sterile was assuming there was contact for thirty seconds with a 90% alcohol-containing sanitizer. Enjoy that salad, playgroup moms!

Clean

adjective
[klēn]

Free from dirt, marks, or stains. "The room was spotlessly clean."

Synonyms: washed, scrubbed, cleansed, cleaned, polished, spotless, unsoiled

Merriam-Webster Dictionary

Changing a dirty diaper may be an extreme, but think of how many things you touch that are dirty. Dirty with physical dirt. Or dirty with chemicals you cannot see, like the perfumes Jenny had in her lavender-scented baby wipes. After applying a sanitizer gel or lotion, do you assume you can go eat lunch? Would you eat a lunch prepared by someone who only used a hand sanitizer to clean their hands instead of soap and water?

Sanitizers can quickly reduce the number of germs on hands in many situations. However,

- Sanitizers do not get rid of all types of germs.
- Hand sanitizers may not be as effective when hands are visibly dirty or greasy.
- Hand sanitizers might not remove harmful chemicals from hands like pesticides and heavy metals. (CDC.gov)

The Centers for Disease Control and Prevention, CDC, is a government-run agency with a mission to protect the American people from health threats. The CDC recommends handwashing with soap and water over using hand-sanitizing agents. They state that sanitizers cannot eliminate ALL germs, especially when hands are already covered in grease or dirt. In addition to physical dirt, hand sanitizers are not effective in removing chemicals. Specifically, the CDC mentions hand sanitizers do not remove pesticides or metals. Another very important, maybe even alarming, fact is that sanitizers also do not remove allergens. For example, the proteins found in peanuts that trigger peanut allergies are not washed away or eliminated from your hands after using hand sanitizer. A person eating peanut butter or a handful of peanuts who uses hand sanitizer has a good chance of still having peanut allergens on their hands ... just sterile allergens. Imagine the danger to someone with a significant peanut allergy?

When using hand sanitizer, think about what it is that you are trying to clean from your hands. Is it dirt, chemicals, bathroom residue, or allergens? Remember that sterile does not mean clean and consider what remains on your hands just now in sterile form. Maybe next time take that extra minute and look for the sink and wash with soap and water. Wash the dirt, chemicals, residues, and allergens down the drain instead of having sterile versions of these items still on your hands.

A Shot in the Eye

Jenny had a schedule for every day of the week. As we know, she had weekly playgroups for her toddler, but her other children were also on a schedule. Ronnie, the four-year-old, had preschool three days a week, and Brock was in second grade. As school-age children, they were germ carriers twenty-four seven. Jenny had them sanitize their hands after school and was completely on board with her children using sanitizers at school. In fact, both children had small, cute containers, on clips, attached to their backpacks. Just in case they encountered a germ along the way during their day.

One Wednesday, Jenny was going about her busy day as usual. It was late morning, and she was standing in line waiting to pick up her daughter, Ronnie, from preschool when her cell phone rang. She looked at the number and recognized it as the elementary school. Quickly she picked up to hear the voice of the school nurse. Jenny was expecting to hear that her son had some sniffles or a belly ache. What she heard set her heart racing.

Brock had gym class Wednesdays. On the way to gym class, the children lined up and took a squirt of hand sanitizer before leaving the classroom. They even sang a song, "Line up, take a squirt, everybody wash their dirt." The hand sanitizer was in a big pump-style bottle on the corner of the teacher's desk. Because second graders were giggling and wiggling while in line, Jenny's son pushed down on the pump mechanism and got a little squirt in his eye.

Had the squirt been a hand soap, Brock would have had to flush his eye out with water and went about his day. However, this little seven-year-old got a squirt of a hand sanitizer containing 90% alcohol in his eye. It burned, so he screamed and cried. Immediately, the teacher called the school nurse. The nurse knew to rinse the boy's eye with lukewarm water for about 10–15 minutes, but she also called Jenny to advise her to take her son to an eye doctor. After all, this little boy had gotten a strong alcohol directly in his eye!

The good news was that damage to the eye's deep tissues was uncommon with contact to alcohol, like the alcohol in sanitizers. However, the cornea, the transparent layer of the eye that directed light into the retina, could suffer a chemical burn. Fortunately, in the case of a chemical burn to the cornea, complete recovery was expected without loss or damage of sight. Jenny was consulted by the doctor that children should not be using hand sanitizer without adult supervision. The doctor said that this was not the first case of sanitizer in the eye of a child or adult he had seen. He even had a patient in their thirties that burned 80% of their cornea. Fortunately, over the course of a few weeks, that patient made a full recovery. In his research, the doctor had read studies showing ocular (eye) exposure to hand sanitizers to account for 3,169 cases of children ages 12 and under over a four-year period. (Table 3) The most comprehensive study he had read was over the years of 2011–2014, and hand sanitizers were used much more frequently now in the 2020s. Accidental eye exposure to sanitizer getting into the eyes of children was not uncommon or a new phenomenon, especially with the placement of many dispensers compared to the height of children.

Exposure Data of Alcoholic Hand Sanitizer, Ages 0–12

Exposure Means	Ages 0–5	Ages 6–12
Ingestion	57,825	4,204
Eye/ocular	1,782	1.387
Skin	2,385	180
Inhalation	74	81

Table 3: Data from the National Poison Data System study 2011–2014.

The doctor also made Jenny aware that sanitizer could get into the eye through touch. Jenny was about to say that she had taught her kids to not touch their eyes and face, for the reason of spreading germs, but was interrupted by the doctor. The doctor interrupted her to say he had seen many cases where children and adults used hand sanitizer, then touched their eyes. People automatically touch their eyes to remove a lash, push hair out of the way, when dust gets into the eye, etc. Eyes are touched for a multitude of reasons, and most people do it instinctively, even when hands are damp from sanitizers or other cleaners for that matter.

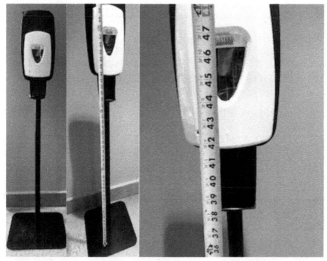

Free-standing hand sanitizer dispenser. Note the location of sanitizer dispensing is waist high for an adult but eye level of a child. (Photo by McEwen)

Jenny, of course, was upset about the sanitizer splash to the eye. However, she saw fault in the process at school, especially the placement of the sanitizer bottle on the teacher's desk, which was eye level of a second grader. When out and about, however, Jenny began to notice that many sanitizer dispensers were at eye level for a child. She saw not only bottles on desks and counters but standing dispensers just inside the doors of stores and even her church. Sometimes there were wall-mounted dispensers in public places. All of these were great to dispense product for an adult whose hands were at waist level, but they were at a dangerous level for children. She was appalled when visiting an office to find a wall dispenser at the same height and next to the elevator call button. Jenny thought of how her kids compete to press the elevator button and how easily they could miss and get a sanitizer squirt on their face or in their eye.

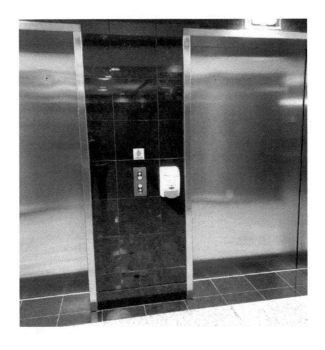

Actual photo of a hand sanitizer dispenser mounted next to an elevator call button. This photo is taken in an office building housing a daycare. (Photo by McEwen)

So, Jenny made a mental note to teach her kids, and her friends, the dangers of these sanitizer dispensers and getting sanitizer in eyes. She also would use her unfortunate experience as an example to talk to the school administration about bottles of hand sanitizer sitting on counters and desks where little eyes were at equal height. Maybe she would take the phrase "use under adult supervision" more seriously.

Don't Drink to That!

One afternoon, while Jenny's son, Brock, was in school and Harper was taking a nap, Jenny had Ronnie do a little quiet time in her room. For quiet time, Jenny's daughter took her little school backpack and said she was going to look at her book she brought home from preschool. After some time, Jenny realized her daughter was awfully quiet, which was not always good. Jenny went to Ronnie's room and found her lying oddly in the middle of the floor, the little girl's hair out in all directions around her. Jenny's pulse quickened. She called to Ronnie with no answer. She lightly rocked Ronnie back and forth. Ronnie was unresponsive. Then Jenny noticed an open, partially empty, bottle of hand sanitizer that had been clipped to the backpack. In a panic, Jenny called 911.

Jenny told the operator she thought her daughter drank hand sanitizer. It appeared she only drank a little bit, but something was wrong. Ronnie was breathing but limp. The paramedics arrived, and Ronnie was taken to the ER where her blood alcohol level was very high and her glucose (sugar) levels were very low. Her daughter was in a coma. The little girl was put on IV fluids, and her blood sugar levels were checked regularly. Thankfully, by the next morning, her blood alcohol levels had dropped and her glucose levels had come back to normal. Jenny was grateful to be able to take her little girl home.

What happened? Jenny thought back through the event and talked at length with the medical staff. Jenny's daughter ingested a 90% alcohol hand sanitizer, only a few little capfuls. Jenny had talked to her kids about how to use hand sanitizer. She had explained that sanitizer was to make germs go away from your hands. Jenny was certain she had told her children not to drink it. She assumed the taste must be terrible. But her daughter had begged for the little bottle that smelled like peaches. Jenny remembered her daughter begging, "Please, Mom, it smells yummy?" Was her daughter drunk? Sort of.

Children do not process alcohol the way adults do. Instead, children's blood glucose (sugar) levels drop, a condition called hypoglycemia. Low blood sugar levels in children can be dangerous and cause seizures, brain injury, or unconsciousness. Hypoglycemia can lead to coma and even death. Low blood sugar dangers are in addition to alcohol poisoning.

Sadly, doctors told Jenny that her daughter was not the first case of hand sanitizer ingestion they had seen or read about. Jenny was referred to several articles to read on data from the FDA and CDC about sanitizer ingestion. Doctors have seen cases of alcohol poisoning due to ingestion in all ages of children. It only takes a few squirts to be the equivalent of a shot or two of hard liquor. Yes, a few squirts are equal to a shot or two. Parents will lock liquor cabinets, yet they do not have any problem sending their kids to school with hand sanitizer linked to their backpacks on a cute little hook. And the sanitizer can be twice as potent as drinking alcohol. That is like a parent sending a small bottle of whiskey to school!

Graph 1 compares the amount of alcohol in hand sanitizer compared to other common liquors. Alcohol content can vary per brand in both hand sanitizers and liquors. In comparison, hand sanitizer has, in many cases, twice as much alcohol as the items locked in liquor cabinets and lockable refrigerators.

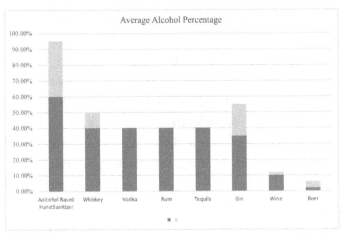

Graph 1. Average alcohol content as a percentage of hand sanitizer versus common liquors. Some alcohols, including hand sanitizer, have a range of alcohol content dependent on brand as shown by the shaded area on the graph.

The FDA classifies alcohol-containing hand sanitizers as over-the-counter drugs. Over-the-counter drugs are medicines that do not require a prescription. Medicines like pain relievers, cough medicines, and allergy pills are examples of over-the-counter drugs. Children are not permitted to take pain relievers or cold medicines to school in their backpacks or bags. Even cough drops must be cleared by the school nurse. But it is common to see small children carrying and using hand sanitizer in schools or on their busses.

SANITIZER

Many hand sanitizers come in brightly colored bottles, can be laced with glitter, and smell like food or candy. This type of packaging makes them very tempting to young children. While a child who licks a tiny amount of hand sanitizer off of his or her hands is unlikely to become sick, a child ingesting any more than a taste of hand sanitizer could be at risk for alcohol poisoning.

The amount of alcohol in hand sanitizer ranges from 40% to 95%. Most hand sanitizer products contain over 60% ethyl alcohol, a stronger alcohol concentration than most hard liquors. By comparison, wine and beer contain about 10–15% and 5–10% alcohol, respectively. Even a small amount of alcohol can cause alcohol poisoning in children. Alcohol poisoning can cause confusion, vomiting, and drowsiness, and in severe cases, respiratory arrest and death.

As of December 31, 2020, poison control centers have managed 24,802 exposure cases about hand sanitizer in children 12 years and younger. (American Association of Poison Control Centers)

The most alarming numbers are data compiled by the CDC from the National Poison Data System 2011–2014. In those years, there were 57,825 cases of ingestion of alcohol-containing hand sanitizers in children ages 0–5. In the age group 6–12, there were 5,681 cases. Yet look around at all the little ones using alcohol-based sanitizers, carrying them to school, and using the automated dispensers. In just the year 2020, hand sanitizer sales increased 600%. Imagine if the childhood ingestion data increased 600%. At that rate, the age group 0–5 would have 289,125 ingestion cases and the ages 6–12 would have 28,405 ingestions. Even scarier, during the COVID-19 pandemic in 2020, the FDA warned that some manufacturers skipped the step of denaturing, which makes for a less appealing taste, all for the sake of more production in less time. (The specifics of denaturing will be discussed in the next chapter.)

Exposure Data of Children Over a 4-Year Period

Year	Number of Exposures
2011	15,971
2012	16,571
2013	16,423
2014	16,328
Total	65,293

Table 4: Number of exposures to alcohol-based hand sanitizers of children ages 0–12 years old reported to poison control centers during the years of 2011–2014.

Hand sanitizers can be up to 95% alcohol. Vodka is approximately 40% alcohol. Think about the adults and children, small children, that rub hand sanitizer on their hands several times a day. In defense, hand sanitizers have at least 5% of other ingredients that make them taste terrible and discourage ingestion. However, it does not take long in stores to see the shelves full of various types of hand sanitizers having options of "scented" like strawberry, citrus, or peach just to name a few. The smell alone can be intriguing to a little one, and it does not take much at a level of 60–95% alcohol to induce alcohol poisoning in a small 30-pound child. Parents may think their child would never ingest something as disgusting as hand sanitizer, but then again, look at how many kids eat paste and boogers.

Remember how hand sanitizer can be up to 95% alcohol? Vodka is approximately 40% alcohol. Would you rub your children's hands in vodka several times per day?

Another note about ingestion of alcohol-based hand sanitizers is the type of ingestion for the children ages 6–12. Although the number of accidental ingestions decrease in this age group, many of the recorded poisonings are from intentional ingestion. Yes, children that young are trying to drink the alcohol not realizing young bodies are affected differently than adults by alcohol consumption. In addition to intentional ingestion being a problem is the possibility of drug interaction with ingestion. Many kids are on medications such as those for attention deficit or hyperactivity or depression.

Poor Jenny has had a few difficult parenting accidents. When she looked back, she realized that in trying to keep her children from getting sick, her daughter almost died of alcohol poisoning and her son could have damaged his eyes. The data she read was mind-blowing. Was concern about bacteria worth damaging one's sight? After all, it was not the sanitizer's fault but Jenny's habits to use the product so frequently. And Jenny's decision to keep sanitizers so readily available. Jenny was starting to realize that germs might not be so bad. Jenny reconsidered what she believed as keeping her family healthy. She thought about her conversations with the medical staff about really keeping sanitizers under adult supervision. After all, she would never allow her children to be around medicines and alcohols. Maybe a little dirt and germs were not so bad. She vowed to start a new habit and promote handwashing with soap and water, while using items like hand sanitizer gels and wipes only when needed, under strict supervision, especially for her children. Maybe she was washing her family sick.

A Little Bit About Alcohol

One summer on the news, Jenny heard that some types of alcohols in hand sanitizers were being banned for purposes of toxicity. Toxicity!!! Toxicity was synonymous with poisonous. Jenny thought she was cleaning germs away, and now she might have been rubbing her hands with toxins in the form of toxic alcohol! Jenny never paid attention to what alcohol type was in her sanitizers. As long as the label on the bottle stated, "kills 99.9% of germs," Jenny bought it! Since she has been an avid user of the products, she did a little research of her own about sanitizers and alcohols. She studied which alcohol types to look for and which alcohol types to avoid. Jenny now paid particular attention to the alcohol types so she could make sure she did not have any with toxic types of alcohol. She was grateful her little Ronnie did not ingest a toxic alcohol.

Jenny's research showed there were four types of alcohol that have been used in hand sanitizers.

A) Isopropyl Alcohol
B) Methanol
C) Ethanol
D) 1-Propanol

Isopropyl alcohol, choice A, is also known as rubbing alcohol. This is the alcohol commonly used prior to injections or having blood drawn. It is a great disinfectant but very drying to the skin. Isopropyl alcohol is not toxic to the skin; however, it loses some of its effectiveness when mixed with aloe, a common advertised moisturizing ingredient in gel sanitizers.

Methanol, choice B, is wood alcohol. Methanol is known to be toxic when absorbed through the skin. Absorption of methanol can cause seizures, permanent blindness, and vomiting. In rare instances, children have died from ingesting methanol-based hand sanitizer. Toxicity from methanol can also occur from absorption through the lungs by inhaling fumes.

In 2020, when the coronavirus pandemic was in full swing and sanitizers were in high demand, the Food and Drug Administration, FDA, banned about 170 brands of hand sanitizer because they contained methanol. Besides cleaning hands, alcohol became a drug of desperation during this pandemic, and people were drinking their sanitizers. Those containing methanol were making people extremely sick and, in some instances, causing death.

With high demand and usage of hand sanitizer in 2020, the FDA reported the following warning about methanol in hand sanitizers:

Consumers who have been exposed to hand sanitizer containing methanol should seek immediate treatment, which is critical for potential reversal of toxic effects of methanol poisoning. Substantial methanol exposure can result in nausea, vomiting, headache, blurred vision, permanent blindness, seizures, coma, permanent damage to the nervous system or death. Although all persons using these products on their hands are at risk, young children who accidentally ingest these products and adolescents and adults who drink these products as an alcohol (ethanol) substitute, are most at risk for methanol poisoning.

Ethanol, choice C, is commonly called ethyl alcohol. What is interesting is ethyl alcohol is also the alcohol in beer, wine, and liquor. There is a difference though between the ethanol we drink and the ethanol we have in topical products. The difference is "denaturing." Denaturing alcohol is the process of adding a chemical to make the alcohol bad-tasting, foul-smelling, and/or poisonous. The ethanol itself is not chemically changed. Therefore, hand sanitizer is like diluted grain alcohol with added chemicals to make it not taste good.

Denature

verb
de·na·ture | [dē-ˈnā-CHər]

To deprive of natural qualities: change the nature of: such as to make (alcohol) unfit for drinking (as by adding an obnoxious substance) without impairing usefulness for other purposes

Synonyms: convert, mutate, reconstruct

Merriam-Webster Dictionary

Another interesting note is the difference between choices B and C, methanol and ethanol. Remember chemistry and the periodic table? Carbon is the sixth element listed on the periodic table. Just one of those little "C" elements present or not makes the difference between the extreme poison option of methanol and the fit for human consumption ethanol.

Then there is choice D, 1-propanol. 1-Propanol is created during fermentation processes and used as a solvent, but it is also used as a disinfectant. 1-Propanol is extremely toxic and sometimes not printed on the label. The FDA called 1-propanol "toxic and life-threatening when ingested."

The FDA reported in 2020 the following about 1-propanol:

> Young children who accidentally ingest these products and adolescents and adults who drink these products as an alcohol (ethanol) substitute are most at risk. Ingesting 1-propanol can cause central nervous system (CNS) depression, which can result in death. Symptoms of 1-propanol exposure can include confusion, decreased consciousness, and slowed pulse and breathing. Animal studies indicate that the central nervous system depressant effects of 1-propanol are 2 to 4 times as potent as alcohol (ethanol). Consumers who have been exposed to hand sanitizer containing 1-propanol and are experiencing symptoms should seek immediate

care for treatment of toxic effects of 1-propanol poisoning. Skin or eye exposure to 1-propanol can result in irritation, and rare cases of allergic skin reactions have been reported.

Prior to FDA warnings, hand sanitizer could contain one or more of the alcohols A–D. When in doubt, pick C, ethanol for cleaning and disinfecting. Just keep in mind that sanitizers are denatured ethanol and contain added chemicals. These added chemicals are what make sanitizers toxic and not intended for human consumption.

After all Jenny has learned about the alcohols in hand sanitizer, she was even more conscious to keep these disinfecting agents away from her children. She was so grateful little Ronnie did not ingest a sanitizer containing methanol. And she realized that even though ethanol-based sanitizers are denatured to discourage ingestion, children may still try them. Jenny was starting to wonder if there was any good from these products.

Washing Ourselves Sick

The Rebuttal

So far, this seems to be a book against the use of hand sanitizers. Not necessarily true. This book is about the overuse and accidental use of hand sanitizers and other disinfecting products, which we will get to in the next chapters. Remember that the overuse and accidental use, not the use, is our focus. This book is not intended to harm the sanitizer industry like Ralph Nadar ruined the Chevrolet Corvair!* If you are going to be around hand sanitizers everywhere, it's good to know as much as possible about what you are putting on your skin and the little hands of your children. Jenny likes the old adage of "learn something every day," so here is a little history on these popular liquids and gels.

The concept of hand sanitizer has been around since the late 1800s. There are records of German surgeons using alcohol-based solutions for their hands. However, the hand sanitizer we know today is credited to a couple, Goldie and Jerry Lippman. They created a waterless cleaner in 1946 for rubber plant workers to remove chemicals from their hands. Goldie worked in the rubber plant. Plant workers used benzene to remove black carbon residue from their hands. Together, Goldie and Jerry created a product called

Gojo, from their names Goldie and Jerry. They mixed the first batch of their Gojo product in the washing machine of Goldie's parents' house. Jerry salvaged pickle jars from local restaurants to package their product and sold door to door to automobile mechanics. Their product was a combination of petroleum jelly, mineral oil, and less than 5% alcohol. Gojo is still used by mechanics today to clean oil and dirt from their hands.

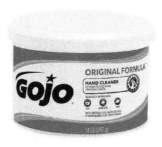

Image from Amazon.com

The Gojo product became a family industry, which later became the basis for the commonly known hand sanitizer Purell. Purell was created in 1988 for use by healthcare workers when soap and water were not available. The appeal of Purell is there is no greasy feel or white residue left behind. You know those bubbles in the bottles that are stuck within the gel? Interestingly, those bubbles actually helped sales. The gel consistency led to those bubbles being suspended in the sanitizer, seen within the bottle, which made the product visually appealing. Hard to believe, but for the first decade of existence, Purell was a money-losing product. Gel-based sanitizers for the general public were new and not well accepted.

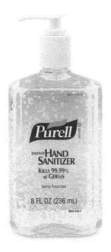

"In 1988, we invented PURELL® Hand Sanitizer, creating a new way for employees, patrons, students, teachers, and everyone else to clean their hands away from the sink, help reduce germs that can cause illness."

GOJO US: History
www.gojo.com/en/About-GOJO/History

Gojo Industries saw a 600% increase in the sales of hand sanitizers during the year 2020. This may have been a pandemic year, but they do not expect the demand to decrease. The company believes the pandemic to be a "wake-up call" that people need to keep themselves clean. In context of the increase in misuse of sanitizers, the makers of Purell have stated publicly that they denature their hand sanitizer for the purpose of preventing misuse such as ingestion.

There is speculation that the creation of hand sanitizer for medical workers and the general public created the attitude of the "germaphobe," one who fears germs. The concept of being able to clean one's hands at any time put the idea into one's head that germs were being picked up on surfaces anytime something was touched. With the availability and portability of hand sanitizers, people could disinfect themselves anytime, anywhere. A great concept when needed. The point is how much and how often is really needed. Picking up germs anytime, anywhere is true. After all, germs are everywhere. Just keep in mind that many germs are not harmful, some may be helpful, and the damage may be more harmful than good.

(*Ralph Nader (1934–present) is an American politician and political activist. Nader authored a book entitled *Unsafe at Any Speed* about the dangers in the automotive industry. In his book, he highly criticized the Chevrolet Corvair as being unsafe. This publication ultimately put an end to Corvair production. The book's criticisms of the car were then proved false.)

Toxins and Chemicals and Residue . . . Oh My!

Let's get back to Jenny. At the end of the grading period, Jenny had an appointment at the elementary school for Brock's school conference. She entered the classroom and took a seat on one of the little second-grade chairs opposite the teacher. Jenny hardly fit on the tiny chair, and she laughed because her knees were up to her chest. Papers of progress reports were passed back and forth across the little classroom table. Jenny noticed the papers did not slide well, but she did not give it another thought. After receiving many compliments on her wonderful son, Jenny got up from the tiny chair and noticed the chair seemed a little sticky. Almost like a film was on the chair. Jenny thought the chair needed a good cleaning.

The following Sunday, Jenny and her family attended Sunday Mass. As her family filed into the pew, Jenny realized she could not slide across the pew like she usually did. The pew looked like there was a little film layer on the wooden surface. Jenny remembered a similar situation at Brock's school and had a realization.

Many institutions such as schools, churches, stores, etc. are deep cleaned on a regular basis to keep free of bacterial and viral outbreaks. A deep clean being a complete wipe down of every surface as much as possible with a disinfectant. The pin pads at checkout lines are wiped between customers, the church pews are cleaned between services, and schools are sanitized at least once a week. Yes, Jenny thinks of all the disinfecting she focuses on, but now she thinks of the big picture and this film layer she is noticing. That film layer is from chemical cleaners that have been wiped on, and wiped on, and wiped on, but never rinsed back off. In other words, layer upon layer of chemical residue. As she slid the papers across the table in the second-grade classroom, Jenny realized the papers were getting stuck on dried chemicals. As she slid across the church pew, her bottom got stuck on dried chemicals. Now she thinks of all the things she touches, things that have been "cleaned," and realizes her hands are picking up dried chemicals. She thinks of her average day. Her pants are getting residue of dried chemicals on chairs, her food is getting dried chemicals from the spraying of grocery carts, and her hands are getting chemical residue from the constant cleaning of keypads and door handles. The grocery cart really sticks with her as she always waits until they are sprayed before taking a cart from the cart corral, then puts her food in that cart! Dried chemicals are getting on her food! The worst she can think of, however, is her children at school, exposed to dried chemicals on every desk, doorknob, cafeteria table, railing . . .

Jenny has often thought about the fumes from some of her cleaners. Sometimes when she sprays down her shower, she accidentally inhales spray mist and coughs, wondering what she is inhaling. She has often thought about the toxicity of chemicals on her skin and usually wears rubber gloves when cleaning her house. Even Jenny thinks about her own cleaning habits and thinks she is covering all the bases of toxic exposure, but rarely does she rinse her cleaners. She had not ever considered chemical residue. Things are often cleaned but not rinsed.

She sprays her counter with disinfectant cleaner and wipes. She sprays her kitchen or bathroom sink and wipes. She mops her floors with floor cleaner. In each cleaning episode, the cleaners are wiped away, but the surface is still wet. Wet with what? Wet with the cleaner that dries leaving residue of which the cleaning products are made. In other words, chemical residue remains all over Jenny's house.

Cleaning supplies, even hand sanitizers, have labels about usage, storage, and contact to skin or ventilation needed during use. Jenny thinks about these labels but thinks she uses these cleaners so quickly that her exposure is extremely limited. And Jenny is just thinking in the present, in other words, chemicals while she is using the product, not the dried chemicals left behind after surfaces dry.

Jenny is a label reader, so she always assumed she purchased cleaners and disinfectants with low levels of toxicity. However, the scariest part of chemical exposure in cleaning products is that the law does not require manufacturers to list all of the ingredients on the labels of consumer products. And the term "green" does not indicate safer. In reference to cleaning supplies, "green" just means safer for the environment in reference to pollution or contamination. Sometimes "green" is referring only to the packaging or the resources used to make the product. Although "green" usually coincides with less toxic, it does not mean nontoxic.

The law does not require manufacturers to list all of the ingredients on the labels of consumer products.

Perfumes are often added to cleaning products and sanitizers as well. Remember Jenny's daughter ingesting the peach-scented sanitizer? Perfumes are just chemical mixtures added to cleaning agents, most notably laundry detergent, and have been known to cause respiratory irritation, headaches, sneezing, and even trigger asthma and allergy reactions. Shockingly, the National Institute of Occupational Safety and Health Administration (OSHA) found that one-third of the fragrance compounds are actually toxic! Even more surprising, perfumes and fragrances are often considered "trade secrets," and manufacturers do not need to list their ingredients. The label stating "fragrance" is acceptable as an ingredient.

The EPA, Environmental Protection Agency, has defined the various types of cleaning products.

Cleaners – Remove dirt through wiping, scrubbing, or mopping.

Sanitizers – Contain chemicals that reduce, but do not necessarily eliminate, micro-organisms such as bacteria, viruses, and molds from surfaces.

Disinfectants – Contain chemicals that destroy or inactivate microorganisms that cause infection. (www.osha.gov)

These definitions are to aid in choosing the appropriate product for the task at hand.

OSHA has developed parameters for protection of workers using chemical cleaners. Parameters such as training for proper use and handling and protective equipment needed when using chemical cleaners. However, the average person, like Jenny, does not know these handling suggestions and may assume that if the product is sold at the local grocery store, it cannot be that toxic.

The amount of data on chemicals in cleaning products and cancers, asthma, allergies, headaches, eye irritation, and skin rashes are vast. (In fact, this list and its details could be its own book.) To summarize, there are eighteen toxic chemicals commonly found in everyday cleaning products. This list of eighteen chemicals has been published with their corresponding commonly caused symptoms (Table 5).

18 Toxic Chemicals Found in Common Cleaning Products

	Chemical	Dangers of Toxicity
1	Alcohol	Headaches, vomiting, nausea, blindness, death; long-term exposure cancers
2	Ammonia	Irritant of eyes, nose, and lungs; can cause skin rashes and burns; extremely poisonous mix with ammonia
3	Bleach	Skin irritant; extremely poisonous mixed with ammonia
4	Butyl Cellosolve	Absorbed through skin causing liver, blood, kidney, and nervous system damage
5	Carbolic Acid (Phenol)	Skin burns and hives; ingestion causes convulsions and possible death

6	Cresol	Burning and numbing of skin; diarrhea, vomiting, headaches; liver, kidney, and lung damage
7	Formaldehyde	Suspected carcinogen; headaches, nausea, eye and nose irritation; ingestion can cause death
8	Glycols	Some are toxic, causing damage to kidneys, liver, and nervous system; some are irritants to eyes, nose, and throat
9	Hydrocarbons (Petroleum Distillates)	Wide range with some being irritants; all are toxic if ingested
10	Acids; Hydrochloric and Phosphoric	Skin burns, blindness; irritant to eyes, nose, and throat
11	Hydrofluoric Acid	Painless absorption through skin into bone
12	Lye (Sodium Hydroxide)	Can dissolve skin; blindness if splashed into the eye; toxic vapors

13	Napthalene	Toxic to inhale; headaches, vomiting; extremely toxic to children
14	Paradichlorobenzenes (PDCBs)	Toxic to inhale; irritant to eyes and nose
15	Perchloroethylene	Dizziness and nausea; liver, nervous system damage; suspected carcinogen
16	Propellants (Propane, Butane and Chlorofluorocarbons)	Irritant to throat, nose, and lungs; regular inhalation can cause death
17	Sulfuric Acid	Skin burns and blindness; toxic to inhale
18	Tricholorethylene (TCE)	Irritant to eyes and nose

Table 5: List of 18 toxic chemicals in common cleaning products and toxic symptoms. Symptoms listed are most common, other symptoms are possible.

This list is published in reference to exposure to chemicals in cleaning products. Of the 18, take formaldehyde, a chemical we associate with preserving scientific specimens and used in embalming fluid. Surprisingly, this same formaldehyde is often in detergents, polishes, and even in things like plastics, mattresses, and plywood.

An example of how these chemicals are present and appear to be harmless is a scented mask-deodorizing spray advertised during mask-wearing mandates of the COVID pandemic. A prominent store display of a major grocery chain displayed several fragrances of mask-deodorizing spray. Right on the front of the brightly colored bottle is "deodorizes mask . . . spray on mask as many times as needed . . . clean formula." The scent choices were citrus or peppermint. That sounds glorious, walk around and smell peppermint instead of coffee breath! And the bottle states "clean formula," which must mean it's healthy or at least not bad for you. Wrong! On the reverse side of the bottle is the list of ingredients with the third ingredient being butylene glycol. (See glycols listed on the list of 18 toxic chemicals.) A quick Google search tells that butylene glycol can be irritating to the skin, eyes, and lungs. Yet the product is created and advertised to spray on an item that touches your face and covers your mouth and nose!

When looking up this product online and reading reviews, there are many reviews stating how lovely it makes the facemask smell. In the product reviews is even a review stating the buyer's mask smells so good they are ordering more for their kids. In other words, ordering more chemicals for your kids to inhale that may irritate their eyes, lungs, and skin. This is just one example of toxic chemicals being in products used regularly and how, unless we look, we are exposing ourselves to potentially toxic chemicals. Imagine going through all the products in the cleaning aisle.

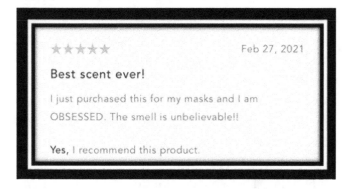

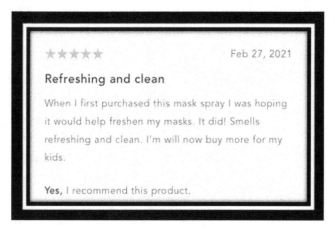

Copies of actual customer reviews about mask-deodorizing spray containing butylene glycol. Butylene glycol can be irritating to eyes,

lungs, and skin, yet these reviews show people inhaling the chemical "scent" and even purchasing the product for their children to inhale.

These are the chemicals that are drying on surfaces—kitchen counters, grocery carts, pin pads—that are then touched by our hands, clothing, and groceries. These are the chemicals that, in dry form, can become airborne and inhaled, aggravating asthma and allergies. In reference to earlier in this book, cleaning with a hand sanitizer is not washing away these chemicals and may be contributing to the residue. Even more surprising is that chemical residue can become a food source for some types of bacteria. Yes, the cleaning product residue can be like a smorgasbord for new germs!

In addition to cancers and respiratory problems, there are chemicals in cleaning products that contribute to hormone disruption. Here is where we make note that some detergents and cleaners can mimic the hormone estrogen, which may promote breast cancer cell growth. Also, these hormone-disrupting chemicals can interfere with the body's natural messaging system and hinder sperm counts. There are even specific chemicals in hand sanitizers that have been shown to have an impact on fertility in mice. Data on fertility with humans and hand sanitizer use is not yet available.

If you don't mind eating anything on the list of ingredients, then the product is

much less likely to have unexpected side effects.

There are chemical cleaners out there that claim to be natural, without harmful vapors and without leaving behind chemical residue. These are all great claims, but a good standard is if you do not mind eating anything on the list of ingredients, then the product is much less likely to have unexpected side effects.

Go back and think about Jenny at the fast-food restaurant with her toddler. The table was smeared and wiped but never rinsed. Those chemicals used to denature the alcohol in the sanitizer remained on the table surface. Those chemicals became residue that stuck to the cheese and grapes. Little Harper had a delicious lunch of chicken, grapes, cheese, and chemicals.

The Memory Is the First To Go

Caroline is Jenny's good friend from college. Actually, the two ladies were not only friends but also roommates. They had completely different majors. Jenny was in marketing and Caroline was a molecular biology major, but they shared the room, shared the same friends, and shared a lot of fun. Also, they shared the same birthday month, which became the perfect excuse to get together once a year to catch up. Although, with their busy lives, occasionally two years would go by without seeing each other, so there was always a lot of catching up to do. One Friday in May, the ladies had a lunch date as Jenny was able to get a sitter for a few afternoon hours. Jenny was going to be late. She texted Caroline to say, "running late, traffic is ridiculous." However, what Jenny actually typed into her phone is "runing late, traffic is rediculous." What happened between Jenny's thumbs pressing the touch screen buttons and the message being sent? The message was being fixed by the miraculous feature called autocorrect.

When Jenny finally arrived, the friends hugged, sat, and began chatting at an alarming pace. Despite the emergencies with her children, whom she now supervised using hand sanitizers, Jenny pulled out her hand sanitizer and sanitized her hands prior to lunch. She offered some to Caroline, who somewhat respectfully declined saying, "No thanks, I don't use hand sanitizer." That response sparked Jenny and Caroline to get into an in-depth conversation about hand sanitizers, which led to a conversation about antibacterial products, which led to a conversation about the immune system. Jenny was starting to lose interest in the discussion. Caroline decided to explain her point using an analogy to Jenny and texting.

Remember Jenny's text about being late and the feature called autocorrect? If Jenny misspells a word, this feature will correct the spelling without Jenny taking a moment to notice her error or even think about the mistake. Similarly, there is spell check for Jenny's emails. Jenny has noticed over the years since the invention of autocorrect and spelling checking software that she has become lax in her spelling of words. Sometimes, she does not even look at what she has typed, assuming the electronic device will fix her spelling. As a result, Jenny does not feel she has as good of spelling skills as she used to. If Jenny needs to spell a word, she must pause and really think about it, sometimes even typing the wrong spelling of the word into a text or email to see if the word gets automatically corrected.

Unbeknownst to Jenny, her immune system and response to germs are similar to the brain and spelling. *Immunological memory* is the term given to the memory of your immune system, and it may be the most important aspect of the immune system. This term means that once you are exposed to a bacteria or virus, your body remembers what that germ looked like. Therefore, if you encounter the bacteria or virus again, your body can fight off the germ faster and more efficiently. It is just like watching a scary movie for the second time, you know where the scary parts are, and they are not so frightening the second time around!

Immunological memory may be the most important aspect of the immune system.

Immunological memory is the basis behind vaccination. Think of a vaccine like an imitation bacteria or virus. A vaccine triggers the immune system to make a response specific to the virus or bacteria imitated in the vaccine. The body responds by building a defense against the vaccine, then files away the defense methods much like putting a recipe into a recipe box. When the real virus or bacteria is encountered, the immune system has the appropriate defenses on file, much like retrieving a recipe. Exposure to things like viruses and bacteria is like natural vaccination.

Since Jenny was so concerned with eliminating germs from her life, her immune system was not making memories. This might seem like a nonissue, but remember that germs are everywhere. Jenny herself will encounter these germs one day or another, maybe when she is older. Or maybe, hopefully not for Jenny's sake, when she is immunocompromised from another infection or even undergoing chemotherapy treatment.

Her body will be weaker than it was in her 30s and less able to fight infection. More importantly, if never exposed, her immune system will not be able to go back into the memory banks and quickly pull up the appropriate recipe for response.

Jenny loves to think she is building a lifetime of wonderful memories for her and her family. She just does not realize she is neglecting her immune system. The immune system wants to make memories too.

Just an Educated Guess

Jenny and Jake have date night. Remember Jake, Jenny's husband? There has been so much focus on the kids we almost forgot about Jake! For Jenny, date night is a much-needed reprieve from her daily routine. Jenny loves her kids and spending time with them, but a little adult time is always lovely. This date night is being shared with two other couples from Jenny and Jake's neighborhood. All the adults have children roughly the same ages, so they have a lot in common and have become good friends as well as neighbors.

Jenny puts on a nice sweater and jeans and a pair of stylish boots. She is excited for a nice restaurant and adult conversation. The evening only gets as far as appetizers when the adult conversation turns into topics about the kids. One of the friends' children, also a boy classmate of Brock, was just diagnosed with asthma, a condition where airways narrow making it difficult to breathe. The boy complained of having breathing problems when playing sports, worse in the spring when trees were blooming. The parents do not want asthma to slow down or interrupt their active boy, so they are now consumed with research and treatment for their son. One reason for developing asthma is heredity, but the parents find it odd that no one in the family has been known to have asthma, yet their son has developed this condition.

All the adults talk about the various people they know, children and even young or middle-aged adults, that have developed asthma. They all discuss how odd it is that when they were growing up, they hardly knew anyone that had asthma, young or old. The conversation then turns to a similar concept with allergies. So many of their kids' friends have allergies, some serious allergies. One couple even has a neighbor that needs to tell delivery persons not to eat peanut butter then handle their packages. Jenny brings up how she asks parents about allergies when they drop their children off to play. She does not want to serve peanut butter cookies to a child with a nut allergy. Again, the same conversation, how very few kids "back in their day" had allergies. Especially allergies that caused someone to carry a lifesaving medicine like that in an EpiPen. Where did all this allergy and asthma come from in the last generation?

The parents of the asthmatic child speak up and say they have been doing extensive research into asthma causes. They have read some remarkably interesting information and some of it relates to why asthma and allergies are more prevalent today than thirty years ago. There is something called the "hygiene hypothesis."

The hygiene hypothesis was developed in 1989 and is just that, a hypothesis, an educated guess. Scientists and doctors have noted over the past decades that rates of asthma, allergies, inflammatory bowel disease, multiple sclerosis (MS), and other autoimmune diseases have increased in wealthy countries. In this same period, wealthy countries have pushed a more sanitary and sterile environment. Studies have shown there is a correlation between lack of exposure to bacteria and viruses at an early age and development of a healthy immune system.

One of the first researchers of the hygiene hypothesis was a doctor from the University of Munich, Erika von Mutius. To pinpoint the concept behind the hypothesis, she stated the following:

> A child's immune system needs education, just like any other growing organ in the human body. The hygiene hypothesis suggests that early life exposure to microbes helps in the education of an infant's developing immune system. (Erika von Mutius)

Summarizing her statement, if the immune system is not given the chance to react, exercise, or make memories, it may attack the wrong target seeing everyday items as foreign intruders. Such is the case with allergies or autoimmune disorders. Throughout time, the immune system has evolved to be constantly on the defensive. With all the sanitizing and cleaning, the immune system does not have anything to do anymore! Our world is cleaner. Our immune systems have never been so unprepared.

There are many studies in support of the hypothesis. One study suggests that children growing up on farms, exposed to animals and dirt, are less likely to develop allergies and other autoimmune disorders. Similarly, Amish children have been noted to have less autoimmune diseases. Amish children are around animals and participate in tasks such as planting crops or plowing fields by hand or with the help of animals. Another study even suggests that children attending daycares are 35% less likely to develop allergies than kids who stay home, possibly because there is more germ exposure in daycare settings. Data exists that children growing up in environments with high levels of allergens and bacteria are less likely to develop allergies and asthma. These are just some examples of supportive research.

Our world is cleaner.
Our immune systems have never been so unprepared.

Again, this is a hypothesis, an educated guess. Other explanations could be that there have been environmental changes over the past 30–40 years or overall dietary or nutrition changes. In addition, there are new pollutants and lifestyle differences over the past few decades. This data may also be coincidence. By no means should every family run out to get a cat or dog, move to a farm, or decide to life in filth. Nonetheless, it sure sounds like we are washing ourselves sick.

Super What??? Superbugs!!!

With the information and experiences Jenny has had with hand sanitizers and cleaners, she is determined to find out anything else she did not know. She does not need any more surprises or crises. Already, she has cleaned out her closets, drawers, purses, and car of any old bottles of sanitizer that may contain anything except ethanol. She has removed bottles her children can access easily and talked to her friends about what adult supervision using sanitizer really means. She warns her friends and family about sending sanitizer with their children on their backpacks. She has even talked to the school administration that sanitizer bottles be used under strict supervision and not kept where children can squirt themselves. Jenny has reevaluated her cleaning process at home too, rinsing cleaners especially from surfaces where food and little hands may have contact.

She is about to ban all hand sanitizers and chemical cleaners from her daily life, but Jenny still has a hard time giving up the habit. Surely there are no more negatives out there. After all, Jenny still wants to be germ-free. To keep from being surprised by another accident, one evening she does a few quick searches for dangers of hand sanitizers and disinfecting cleaners. She sees articles about alcohol poisoning and chemical residue and harmful vapors, but Jenny also sees a term she is unfamiliar with, *superbugs*. Jenny has no idea what a superbug is, but it does not sound like something she wants or needs, so she delves further into her information search. What she finds is a terrifying concept she has heard before but never gave much thought.

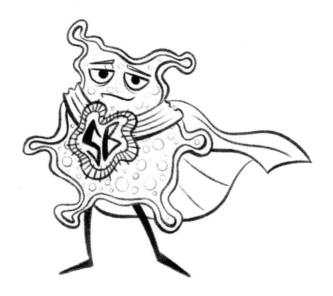

Superbugs are germs, bacteria, and sometimes fungus that have become resistant to antibiotic or antifungal treatment. Overuse of antibiotics is what Jenny learns contributes most to the development of superbugs. Just like Charles Darwin coined the term "survival of the fittest," bacteria (and fungi) are able to undergo random mutation that allows them to survive even under antibiotic treatment. The most common superbug is MRSA (pronounced "mersa"), methicillin-resistant *Staphylococcus aureus*. Jenny has heard of MRSA and knows it's resistant to treatments, but otherwise she is not very familiar. As the name states, this is a bacteria of the "staph" genus. Staph infections are not uncommon. MRSA, as the name implies, has become resistant to methicillin, the common antibiotic used to treat staph infections. Because of its resistance to antibiotics, MRSA can withstand treatment with this common antibiotic and get into the blood stream and spread through the body. Since treatment with antibiotics is difficult and often ineffective, death is a highly possible outcome with MRSA and other superbugs.

Symptoms of infection with an antibiotic-resistant germ look just like other germ infections. A normal course of antibiotics is usually prescribed but fail to be effective. Superbug infections are not diagnosed until routine treatments do not work, and many times the infection has become too advanced for any treatment.

Interestingly, superbugs are not arising only from overuse of prescription antibiotics. There are anti-bacterial agents in many cleaning products. What is the difference between antibiotic and antibacterial? Not much. Antibiotics are medicines that are antibacterials. An antibiotic kills or inhibits the growth of micro-organisms, bacteria, fungi, parasites, etc. The word antibiotic means "against life." Examples of common antibiotics are penicillin and amoxicillin. Antibacterials are agents that kill bacteria, inhibit bacterial growth, or affect the ability of bacteria to reproduce. (see the word "bacteria" in antibacterial). Triclosan is the most common antibacterial. In other words, antibiotics kill microorganisms, and antibacterials kill *only* the microorganism bacteria. Regardless of if antibiotic or antibacterial, they are both targeting bacteria that can become resistant and become superbugs.

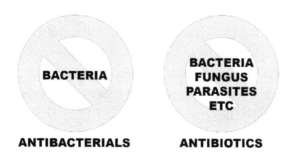

Now Jenny is panicking. She uses antibiotics when she gets sinus infections and other illnesses and is guilty of exaggerating a cold to get a prescription just to alleviate her symptoms more quickly. But she is also constantly spraying household surfaces with antibacterial agents. Even the cleaners not labeled as "antibacterial" are labeled at killing 99.9% of bacteria and viruses, in other words "antibacterial." If overuse of antibiotics can lead to superbugs, imagine the superbug population that could stem from all the antibacterial cleaning agents being used everywhere!

At least, Jenny thinks, her hand sanitizer usage seems to not be contributing to the superbug problem.

Jenny cannot believe what she reads next. There is very little information, but new evidence is showing superbugs may be caused from overuse of hand sanitizer. There is recent evidence that *Enterococcus faecium* is developing alcohol resistance. Yes, resistance to alcohol, the sterilizing agent in hand sanitizers. *Enterococcus faecium* is a bacteria found as a normal inhabitant of the gastrointestinal tract, the gut. Inside the gut these are beneficial bacteria helping with digestion. However, outside the gut these bacteria can cause such things as neonatal meningitis (inflammation of the protective membranes of the central nervous system in young infants) or endocarditis (an infection of the heart's lining). These bacteria are one of the leading causes of infections in hospitals. Due to such frequent use of alcohol-based sanitizers, these bacteria are developing the ability to withstand alcohol and survive on hands cleaned with hand sanitizers.

According to the CDC, more than 2.8 million drug-resistant infections happen yearly in just the United States. Of those, more than 35,000 are fatal. That is a 1.25% death rate once infected. That sounds like a low number, but superbugs can infect anyone. Like with many illnesses, people with weakened immune systems are more likely to become infected by superbugs. However, since superbugs are new versions, or strains, even healthy people are at risk. If the superbug is resistant to common treatments, combined with no previous immune experience, an infected individual can face serious problems.

Jenny has been so concerned about her family's health, constantly scrubbing, wiping, and sanitizing that she never considered the idea that she may be creating or contributing to a new "bug." Not just Jenny alone, but the combination of all the Jennys out there with their attempt at sterile environments are contributing to the creation of superbugs. In the efforts Jenny has taken to keep her family healthy and free of germs, she may be playing a part in creating new bacterial strains that will be detrimental to her children's or grandchildren's lives.

What can be done about superbugs? For starters, antibiotics should only be taken when needed. Many infections can be fought by the immune system. The immune system may take a little longer than an antibiotic, but our own bodies have a great weapon. Maybe more importantly is the fact that the CDC recommends first on the list of preventing a superbug infection washing hands thoroughly with soap and water. This, thinks Jenny, washing with soap and water, is where we are going to start.

Out with the New, In with the Old

When Jenny looks back over the past few months, she cannot believe what has happened to her and her family. Her son getting sanitizer in his eyes could have resulted in permanent eye damage. Her daughter could have died from ingesting a product Jenny gave her as a cute trinket on a backpack hook. And let us not forget that Jenny may have served fecal matter salad to her best friends. All this because she was so concerned about keeping her family healthy. How could she have let all of this happen? How could she have not seen these crises as possibilities? She knew the warnings, but she was too concerned about germs.

Jenny also reflects on her realization that the world around her was disinfecting and cleaning just the same, spraying and wiping but rarely rinsing. Items she and her family touched every day were coated with chemical residue. This residue could be carcinogenic, poisonous, or even more shocking and disgusting, a bacterial food source. And all the while Jenny was thinking "clean." How could she not have thought that constant cleaning of surfaces was not leaving chemical residue on the things she and her family touched? Not to mention the obvious fumes or airborne residue.

Jenny laughs at herself. Jenny is smart. She has a degree in marketing, and she was won over by the marketing techniques and advertisements for these products. She saw TV ads about eliminating bacteria, read magazine articles about keeping children healthy and germ-free, and was constantly faced with prominently located store displays of sanitizing products in bright-colored bottles. Most of these products have warning labels, "not for use on children" or "keep out of reach of children," but Jenny was so concerned with eliminating germs she was not seeing the big picture. After all, she was not spraying her children down head to toe with disinfectant. But the big picture being germs. Bacteria, viruses, and fungi are everywhere, they have been around since before humans, and they are not going away.

Superbug is now a term Jenny understands. She realizes that overcleaning may be just as bad as never cleaning at all. And she understands a little more about her immune system and how important this natural, highly evolved mechanism truly is.

Bacteria, viruses, and fungi are everywhere, they have been around since before humans, and they are not going away.

She has not gone full circle and lives in filth, but she is aware of her cleaning habits. She rinses chemical cleaners when possible, and she has learned to use truly natural cleaners like vinegar, baking soda, and a little elbow grease. Jenny has done her research. Does she still use hand sanitizer? Yes, but as intended when soap and water are not available. She supervises the use of sanitizers with her children.

Jenny has shared her stories and experiences with friends, family, and even on social media with complete strangers. She sees the importance of understanding the amount of alcohol in hand sanitizers and the accidental, or intentional, consequences that can occur. Also, she has spoken to her school district administration advocating for sanitizer bottles and dispensers to be kept truly out of children's reach and for soap-and-water "wash-up" time being given before lunch or snack time. She also had "small bottle of hand sanitizer" removed from the school supply list.

Does Jenny still clean and wipe surfaces in her home? Yes, but she is cognizant of the products she uses. She tries to pay attention to the ingredients in her cleaners. After all, she always carries a smart phone with her, so she can easily look up an ingredient and check the warnings. Occasionally she really does want a good chemical cleaner, like cleaning her shower after her family of five bathes for a week. In that case, Jenny is sure to wipe any residue away or rinse the surface clean.

Is Jenny now living germ-free? No, she has realized germs have been around since the start of life on Earth and are not going anywhere. Humans are not germ-free. Although she will never know, she also must wonder if her children's colds, coughs, runny noses, and sore throats could be a result of under-exposure to germs. In other words, no immunologic memory to call upon. Or if these illnesses could all be a learning process for her children's immune systems. Maybe they all need a little immune system exercise. Jenny and her family are focusing on making their immunologic memory bank while keeping themselves clean not sterile.

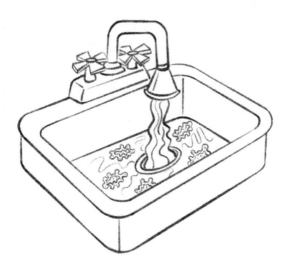

Although maybe not as convenient or taking an extra minute to do, Jenny has pushed for her and her family to prioritize handwashing. Good old soap and water. Germs, dirt, allergens, and chemicals are now going down the drain at Jenny's house instead of building up on surfaces and hands. The skin on their hands is not being dried and cracked allowing the entry of germs like the umbrella without holes keeps you safe from rain. Jenny and her family are now washing away

dirt, chemicals, and germs instead of washing themselves sick.

Getting the Last Word

This book has been about ten years in the making. My first introduction to hand sanitizer was at a fast-food restaurant with a "friend" and her toddler. Yes, the incident in this book was a real occurrence, and I was at the table witnessing the whole thing. I asked my friend what she was doing and was handed the bottle, the first bottle of hand sanitizer I had ever seen. Immediately I was skeptical and realized that 99.9% sanitization still meant 0.1% contamination.

I also witnessed the dirty diaper incident as I was one of the moms at the playgroup. (A special note to my friends, I was in many playgroups over the years.) After this incident, I started to observe what people were doing when using hand sanitizer and what they did after using hand sanitizer. All I could think of was that the dirt, or germs, was still physically present just now sterile.

I have an undergraduate degree in molecular biology/biotechnology and a graduate degree in micro-biology. Germs were my career before I put my career on hold to stay home with my sons, much like Jenny. I have seen those commercials and magazine articles stating or insinuating how everything needs to be disinfected. I have witnessed people using disinfecting products on themselves and even on very young children. The more things I saw, the more I would think and overthink. My biology-based mind would start churning, and I became obsessed.

Often, I would get into discussions and even disagreements with friends and acquaintances about using hand sanitizer. Much like Jenny and Caroline, I would argue the effects on your hands and skin. Mostly, I would argue about the dirt still being on your hands. Usually, people did not have much to respond with other than sanitizing made them feel better and safer. Sometimes people would say they did not like using sanitizers but did anyway, just in case. And often I got the eye roll from friends as I lectured. I did not consider post-hand-sanitizer hands to be clean, or any surface wiped with hand sanitizer for that matter, and I had a tough time letting those thoughts go unspoken.

I then started paying attention to other habits I heard about, like spraying the bottoms of your shoes with Lysol when you enter your home or wiping down grocery cart handles. I thought about how we are stripping ourselves of helpful bacteria in this self-sterilizing process. I have taken note of countless people that follow many sanitizing habits, and the habits never die. It seems they multiply into a bigger sanitizing obsession. Over the years I have noticed that these people are the ones who themselves, or their kids, are so often sick. Coincidence maybe, but in my mind, I attributed these illnesses to lack of germ exposure, lack of immune system exercise.

Since I have children of school age, I am also aware how sanitizers are being used in schools instead of sending kids to the bathroom to "wash up" as I was told as a kid. I witnessed firsthand the pump dispensers on teachers' desks or by the classroom door so kids could "take a pump" before leaving the room. I researched and found stories about children ingesting hand sanitizer because it smelled good. Or using it so much they were getting alcohol poisoning by absorption through their skin. Yet these concepts never crossed parents' minds. When I would bring up these concepts with people, they would laugh. My friends thought I was living in a bacterial-laden world.

I saw how sanitizing was marketed. In shopping for a new dishwasher, the salesman looked at my then young children and said, "This dishwasher has a sanitizing cycle to sterilize your dishes." Of course, my answer was "but when you unload the dishes, you touch every dish and fork and spoon with your hands, so they are no longer sterile." A few years later, I had a similar experience with a washing machine.

The final straw was during the COVID-19 pandemic. Hand sanitizers, cleaners, and disinfecting sprays were flying off the shelves. Many shelves were bare. Any item relevant to cleaning was out of stock. The obsession of sanitizing and overcleaning became a compulsion. A habit that many people acquired and are afraid to discontinue.

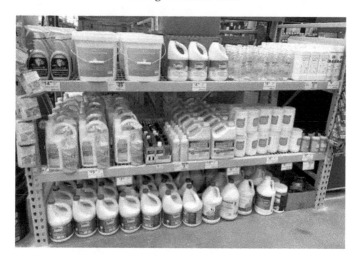

Common end-cap display at a local store showing a multitude of disinfecting supplies. (Photo by McEwen)

During the COVID-19 pandemic, I went to church and tried to slide across the pew. I could not slide. It was then that I realized the pew had been cleaned repeatedly, leaving so much chemical cleaner residue that there was a dried chemical layer on the pew preventing me from sliding across. Those chemicals were probably all over my hands and clothes by the time I left church. Now my brain started to think about all the "deep cleaning" that was happening. In my grocery store, where we purchase the food we eat, employees would walk up and down the freezer section spraying door handles after customers opened doors. Before being returned for use by the next customer, shopping carts were being sprayed with a garden sprayer full of disinfectant and left to air-dry. These dried, and sometimes still wet, chemicals were getting on my hands and groceries. Even worse, in my opinion, the schools where our developing children were sitting, learning, and eating their lunches were "deep cleaning" every few days. Deep cleaning desks, railings, door handles, lunch tables, everything our children touched all day long. And I know the kids are touching their pencils, laptops, phones, etc. that come home and set on the kitchen table for homework. Besides the fact that most kids are probably touching their faces all day long too.

I was never a big label reader, but when I started this book, I began looking at ingredient labels on cleaners. For example, I looked at a label on a fabric sanitizing spray. Directly on the label were warnings about eye irritation and skin contact. Granted, the label is probably talking about getting the actual spray on contact, but this product is also advertised to spray items like stuffed animals to prevent traumatizing your child by putting the stuffed animal into the washing machine. In this instance, the product is not being rinsed. Imagine sending your little one to bed with a stuffed animal coated with a layer of dried chemical with this warning label?

PRECAUTIONARY STATEMENTS: Hazards to Humans and Domestic Animals. CAUTION: Causes moderate eye irritation. Avoid contact with eyes and skin. Wash thoroughly with soap and water after handling and before eating, drinking, chewing gum, using tobacco or using the toilet.

Commercials were prevalent advertising spray to disinfect hard surface floors, disinfect your laundry, disinfect fabric surfaces in your home, and disinfect the air. Companies were even advertising sanitizing the air vents in your home. And not just commercials, every store had displays of assorted items to disinfect everything you could think of.

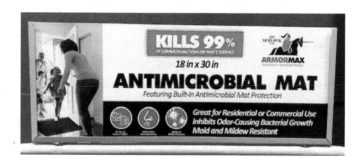

Antimicrobial mat being sold for both residential and commercial use. The mat is intended to sanitize shoe soles when walking across. (Photo by McEwen)

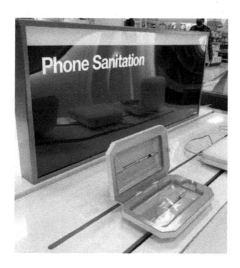

Prominent display of phone sanitation box being sold to sterilize your cell phone. (Photo by McEwen)

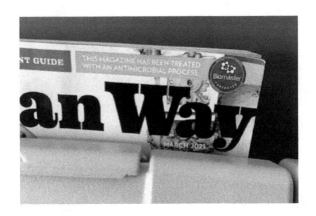

Magazine in the seat pocket of an airplane seat. Magazine is stamped that it has been treated with a silver additive to inhibit growth of bacteria and viruses. (Photo by McEwen)

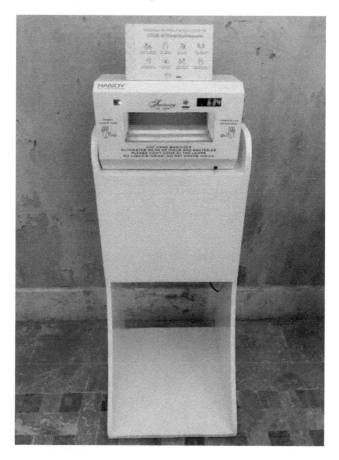

UV hand sanitation station, another way to eliminate bacteria completely from your hands. (Photo by McEwen)

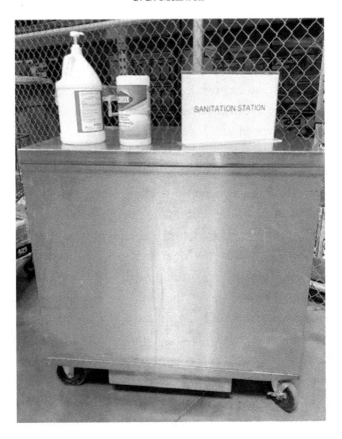

Sanitation station in local warehouse-type store. These stations are placed throughout the store for customer use while shopping. (Photo by McEwen)

Given the deep cleaning everything, leaving dried chemicals everywhere, and the hand sanitizers used excessively, I felt compelled to write this book. In the writing process, I was even more alarmed to learn of alcohol poisoning among children, the fact that allergens like peanut proteins are not removed by hand sanitizers, and that fertility may be affected by hand sanitizer's sterilization. Not to mention the possible link to breast cancer from household cleaning products, a disease so prevalent in my family.

When I came across the information about the hygiene hypothesis, I was obsessed. I was up at 2:00 a.m. reading articles about this hypothesis. "This is what I have been preaching," I thought. I have been conversing this concept of needing exposure to germs and exercising the immune system to friends and family for years. The chapter "The Memory is the First To Go" is mostly my own thoughts. However, the hygiene hypothesis took my thoughts one step further. I had no idea about the link to cleanliness and autoimmune disorders. And I have had countless conversations with friends and family about how many kids have allergies and autoimmune diseases, yet I did not know many kids with these symptoms when I was a kid. Just like Jenny and her friends, I always wondered where all these allergies and other autoimmune conditions came from. Again, it is just a hypothesis—a guess not proven—but it sure is coincidental.

Do I clean? Yes, constantly! However, in writing this book, I am now even more particular when choosing my cleaners. Most of the time I use vinegar diluted in water or even cheap vodka diluted 1:4 in water. I know diluted vodka is an alcohol, but I do not have young children in my home anymore. These two solutions are cheaper than most commercially made cleaners too! Yes, I do use harsh chemicals sometimes. However, when I do, I try to rinse the cleaners to diminish or eliminate any chemical residue left behind. Do I use hand sanitizer? As of the construction of this book, I have used hand sanitizer three times in my life. Every use a result of required use due to office or store policy.

In no way am I against cleaning and disinfecting. I am trying to raise awareness of overcleaning, over-disinfecting, and the use of the chemical-laden products to do these tasks. I had no idea some of these surface sprays contained things so toxic!

When advertisements or talk show hosts are saying things like "germ-free environment," I get nervous. Germs will prevail, no matter how much we clean. And germs will follow the same biological concept as other species, "survival of the fittest," and mutate to withstand the medical treatments we do have. The superbug concept scares me, really scares me. There is belief among the scientific community that the first life form on Earth was a single-celled organism, much like a prehistoric bacteria. Germs, categorizing bacteria and viruses together, have been around millions—yes, millions—of years. They are not going anywhere. We need to learn to be clean, not sterile, and to make a lifetime of memories with our bacterial friends.

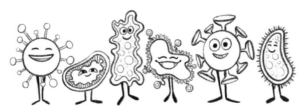

Are you overcleaning and exposing yourself to harsh chemical residues? Are you getting holes in your protective skin umbrella? Are you contributing to the evolution of superbugs? And I will leave you with one final question to ask yourself. Are you washing yourself sick?

Handwashing Day

Shelter Dog Day, Ice Cream Day, Redhead Day, you name it, there is a day for it! In 2008, Global Handwashing Day was first celebrated. To commemorate the day, more than 120 million children around the globe washed their hands with soap and water. Over 70 countries participated. Global Handwashing Day was advocated to spread awareness of using soap and water, demonstrating a simple, effective, and economical way to clean hands in the prevention of disease. The ultimate goal is to save lives. Handwashing Day has also provoked communities to build sinks and other types of wash stations, showing the importance of cleanliness and clean hands using only water and soap. The day is celebrated yearly on October 15.

The Global Handwashing Partnership founded Global Handwashing Day. Celebrated for the first time in 2008 and observed every year on October 15, Global Handwashing Day is to encourage washing hands with soap and water. The day also advocates that handwashing with soap and water is more effective at preventing disease and does not pose the threat to your health that using chemicals and alcohol-based sanitizers cause. (CDC.gov)

In 2020, the theme for Global Handwashing Day was "Hand Hygiene for All." The theme was meant as a reminder of the importance of handwashing with soap and clean water to promote a healthy future.

Acknowledgments

Kraig

Without you, I never would have authored this book.
For years you listened to me lecture about over
sanitizing and immune systems. One day when I said
I should write a book, you pushed me to do just that.
I love you. Thank you.

Alec and Kyle

You two allowed me to have the experiences of
playgroups and schools to notice how sanitizing
products were being used. And, of course, listened to
me tell you not to use hand sanitizer when offered
and tolerated my lecturing about cleaning chemicals. I
love you both and wish you both long, happy, healthy
lives!

Hailey Bair

Thank you for creating the fun drawings in my book,
especially for bringing life to my superbug!

Chrissy and EFC Services, LLC

Thank you for the editing and help with general
writing. I am grateful to have found someone that will
be honest with me and give me ideas at a short notice.

Friends

I wish I could name you all, but there would be a lengthy list. Thank you for listening to me rant about hand sanitizers and cleaning products over lunches and walks. And for some of you giving me sanitizing experiences to think about.

Family

Especially my dad and mom, Dick and Carol. Thank you for having faith in me when I wanted to go to college and major in something you could not pronounce. I hope I make you proud.

About the Author

S.B. McEwen holds a bachelor of science degree in molecular biology/biotechnology from Westminster College and a master's degree in microbiology from Duquesne University. Her graduate research was with E. coli O157:H7. She worked as a molecular biologist in cancer research, diabetes research, and cystic fibrosis research and holds scientific publications in her research areas.

After working in research for approximately eight years, she left her career to raise her two sons. Periodically, she has been an adjunct instructor in biology at a local college. McEwen has volunteered with her local school district's science fair, the high school lacrosse parent boosters, and various other organizations.

She is passionate about science and even bought a microscope for home use to share the microscopic world with her sons.

She lives in western PA with her husband, two sons, and shelter dog. Her family is her primary career.

Email: booksbysbmcewen@hotmail.com
Facebook: www.facebook.com/sb.mcewen
Instagram: @booksbysbmcewen

References

Hmmm . . . Really?

CDC. 2020. "Show Me the Science – When & How to Use Hand Sanitizer in Community Settings." https://www.cdc.gov/handwashing/show-me-the-science-hand-sanitizer.html.

American Association of Poison Control Centers. 2021. "Hand Sanitizer." https://aapcc.org/track/hand-sanitizer.

Fukushima, Kurumi. 2020. "5 Hidden Dangers of Hand Sanitizers." https://www.thestreet.com/markets.

MacPherson, Lynn. 2018. "Allergic Reaction to Hand Sanitizers." https://healthfully.com/allergic-reaction-to-hand-sanitizers.

Taghipour, Delaram. 2020. "More Children Ingesting Hand Sanitizers Due To Manufacturing Lapses: FDA." https://abcnews.go.com/Health/children-ingesting-hand-sanitizers-due-manufacturing-lapses-fda/story?id=70366578.

This is My Friend Jenny

Berger, Jennifer. 2015. "Five Parenting Trends To Watch in 2015." https://www.newsday.com/lifestyle/family.

Smith, Tiffany. 2016. "Care.com's Predictions for the Hottest Parenting Trends in 2015." https://www.care.com/c/stories/4694.

Grapes of Wrath

CDC. 2020. "Show Me the Science – When & How to Use Hand Sanitizer in Community Settings." https://www.cdc.gov/handwashing/show-me-the-science-hand-sanitizer.html.

MacPherson, Lynn. 2018. "Allergic Reaction to Hand Sanitizers." https://healthfully.com/allergic-reaction-to-hand-sanitizers.

Would You Rub Alcohol on Your Heart?

University of Colorado at Boulder. 2010. "New CU-Boulder Hand Bacteria Study Holds Promise for Forensics Identification." https://www.colorado.edu/today/2010/03/15/new-cu-boulder-hand-bacteria-study-holds-promise-forensics-identification.

University of Colorado at Boulder. 2008. "Women Have More Diverse Hand Bacteria Than Men." https://phys.org/news/2008-11-women-diverse-bacteria-men.html.

Bailey, Regina. 2019. "5 Types of Bacteria That Live on Your Skin." https://www.thoughtco.com/bacteria-that-live-on-your-skin.

Byrd, A., Y. Belkaid, and J. Segre. 2018. "The Human Skin Microbiome." *Nature Reviews Microbiology*

16: 143–155.
https://doi.org/10.1038/nrmicro.2017.157.

Curley, Christopher. 2020. "FDA Expands List of Hand Sanitizers That Contain Toxic Methanol."
https://www.healthline.com/health-news/fda-says-avoid-9-hand-sanitizers-that-contain-toxic-methanol.

Korab, Alek. 2020. "9 Side Effects of Using Hand Sanitizer, According to Doctors."
https://www.eatthis.com/side-effects-hand-sanitizer-doctors/.

McInnis, Kaitlyn. 2020. "The Scary Effect Using Too Much Sanitizer Can Have on Your Health."
https://www.theladders.com/career-advice/the-scary-effect-using-too-much-sanitizer-can-have-on-your-health.

Shahi, Surkriti. 2019. "Global Handwashing Day 2019: 5 Side Effects of Hand Sanitizers You Didn't Know About."
https://www.thehealthsite.com/diseases-conditions/global-handwashng-day-1029.

The Dirty Diaper

CDC. 2020. "Show Me the Science – When & How to Use Hand Sanitizer in Community Settings."
https://www.cdc.gov/handwashing/show-me-the-science-hand-sanitizer.html.

Oxford Dictionaries, s.v. "clean," accessed January, 2021.

FARE. 2021. "Cleaning Methods."
https://www.foodallergy.org/resources/cleaning-methods.

Korab, Alek. 2020. "9 Side Effects of Using Hand Sanitizer, According to Doctors."
https://www.eatthis.com/side-effects-hand-sanitizer-doctors/.

MacPherson, Lynn. 2018. "Allergic Reaction to Hand Sanitizers." https://healthfully.com/allergic-reaction-to-hand-sanitizers.

A Shot in the Eye

Au, Sunny Chi Lik. "Hand Sanitizer Associated Ocular Chemical Injury: A Mini-Review on Its Rise Under Covid-19." *Visual Journal of Emergency Medicine* 21: 100881.
https://pubmed.ncbi.nlm.nih.gov/32923696/
.

Duerr, Charlie. 2020. "The CDC Says You Must Keep Hand Sanitizer Away from Kids Under This Age." Retrieved from
https://bestlifeonline.com/hand-sanitizer-kids-cdc/

Hazanchuk, Vered. 2021. "Hand Sanitizer in the Eye: Is It Dangerous?" https://www.aao.ord/eye-heath/tips-prevention.

Lazarus, Russel. 2020. "Eye Emergency: Hand Sanitizer in Your Eye."
https://www.optometrists.org/eye-emergency-hand-sanitizer-in-your-eye/

Letzter, Rafi. 2021. "Hand Sanitizer Is Causing an
    Epidemic of Chemical Burns To Children's
    Eyes." https://www.livescience.com/covid-
    19-pandemic-hand-sanitizer-burns.html.
Santos, C. et al. 2017. "Reported Adverse Health
    Effects in Children from Ingestion of
    Alcohol-Based Hand Sanitizers – United
    States, 2011–2014." http://dx.doi.org/10.

Don't Drink to That

American Association of Poison Control Centers.
    2021. "Hand Sanitizer."
    https://aapcc.org/track/hand-sanitizer.
2020. "Hand Sanitizers: How Toxic Are They?"
    https://www.poisonscontrol.org.
2020. "Hand Sanitizer Market Size, Share & Trends
    Analysis Repot by Product (Gel, Foam,
    Liquid), by Distribution Channel
    (Hypermarket & Supermarket, Drug Store,
    Specialty Store, Online), by Region, and
    Segment Forecasts, 2020–2027."
    https://www.grandviewresearch.com.
CDC. 2020. "Show Me the Science – When & How
    to Use Hand Sanitizer in Community
    Settings."
    https://www.cdc.gov/handwashing/show-
    me-the-science-hand-sanitizer.html.
"Alcohol: A Dangerous Poison for Children."
    https://www.poison.org/articles/alcohol-a-
    dangerous-poison-for-children.

Duerr, Charlie. 2020. "The CDC Says You Must Keep Hand Sanitizer Away from Kids under This Age." https://bestlifeonline.com/hand-sanitizer-kids-cdc/.

Fukushima, Kurumi. 2020. "5 Hidden Dangers of Hand Sanitizers." https://www.thestreet.com/markets.

Gershman, Jennifer. 2017. "3 Things You Should Know about Ingestion of Alcohol-Based Hand Sanitizer." https://www.pharmacytimes.com/view/3-things-you-should-know-about-ingestion-of-alcohol-based-hand-sanitizer.

Goodman, Brenda. 2015. "Hand Sanitizers Poisoning More Kids." https://www.webmd.com/children/news/20150915.

Korab, Alek. 2020. "9 Side Effects of Using Hand Sanitizer, According to Doctors." https://www.eatthis.com/side-effects-hand-sanitizer-doctors/.

Martyn, Amy. 2020. "String of Fatal Poisonings from Ingestion of Toxic Hand Sanitizer Highlights Limits of FDA Powers." https://www.salon.com/2020/10/06/string-of-fatal-poisonings-from-ingestion-of-toxic-hand-sanitizer-highlights-limits-of-fda-powers_partner/.

McInnis, Kaitlyn. 2020. "The Scary Effect Using too Much Sanitizer Can Have on Your Health." https://www.theladders.com/career-advice/the-scary-effect-using-too-much-sanitizer-can-have-on-your-health.

O'Donovan, Anna. 2020. "The Perils and Pitfalls of Hand Sanitizer." https://www.allergystandards.com/news-events/.

Pruitt, Albert. et al. "Ethanol in Liquid Preparations Intended for Children." *Pediatrics* (1984): 405–407.

Santos, C. et al. 2017. "Reported Adverse Health Effects in Children from Ingestion of Alcohol-Based Hand Sanitizers – United States, 2011-2014." http://dx.doi.org/10.

Schneir, A.B, and R.F. Clark. 2013. "Death Caused by Ingestion of an Ethanol-Based Hand Sanitizer." *Journal of Emergency Medicine* 45, no. 3 (September 2013): 358–60. Epub.

Settembre, Jeanette. 2020. "Hand Sanitizer Poisoning During Coronavirus Surges, Calls To Poison Control Up 70%." https://www.foxnews.com/health/hand-sanitizer-poisoning-coronavirus.

Taghipour, Delaram. 2020. "More Children Ingesting Hand Sanitizers Due To Manufacturing Lapses: FDA." https://abcnews.go.com/Health/children-ingesting-hand-sanitizers-due-manufacturing-lapses-fda/story?id=70366578.

Terlep, Sharon. 2021. "Hand Sanitizer Sales Jumped 600% in 2020. Purell Maker Bets Against a

Post-Pandemic Collapse." *The Wall Street Journal*, January 22, 2021.

Yerby, Nathan. 2021. "Types of Alcohol – List of Drinks by Alcohol Content – Alcohol Rehab Guide." https://www.alcoholrehabguide.org/alcohol/types/.

A Little Bit About Alcohol

2020. "Hand Sanitizers: How Toxic Are They?" https://www.poisonscontrol.org

Curley, Christopher. 2020. "FDA Expands List of Hand Sanitizers That Contain Toxic Methanol." https://www.healthline.com/health-news/fda-says-avoid-9-hand-sanitizers-that-contain-toxic-methanol.

Oxford Dictionaries, s.v. "denature," accessed February 12, 2021.

Farber, Madeline. 2020. "New Toxin Found in Certain Hand Sanitizers; FDA Adds Products To 'Do Not Use' List." https://www.foxnews.com/health/new-toxin-found-some-hand-sanitizers-fda.

Martyn, Amy. 2020. "String of Fatal Poisonings from Ingestion of Toxic Hand Sanitizer Highlights Limits of FDA Powers." https://www.salon.com/2020/10/06/string-of-fatal-poisonings-from-ingestion-of-toxic-hand-sanitizer-highlights-limits-of-fda-powers_partner/.

O'Donovan, Anna. 2020. "The Perils and Pitfalls of Hand Sanitizer." Retrieved from https://www.allergystandards.com/news_events/the-perils-and-pitfalls-of-hand-sanitizer/.

Taghipour, Delaram. 2020. "More Children Ingesting Hand Sanitizers Due To Manufacturing Lapses: FDA." https://abcnews.go.com/Health/children-ingesting-hand-sanitizers-due-manufacturing-lapses-fda/story?id=70366578.

The Rebuttal

2020. "History of Hand Sanitizer | Best Practices Guide." http://wholesalehandsanitizers.com/history-of-hand-sanitizer/.

Huddleston, Tom. 2020. "The History of Hand Sanitizer – How the Coronavirus Staple Went from Mechanic Shops To Consumer Shelves." https://www.cnbc.com/2020/03/27/coronavirus-the-history-of-hand-sanitizer-and-why-its-important.html.

https://nader.org/biography

What Doesn't Cause Cancer

2021. "How Toxic Are Your Household Cleaning Supplies?" https://www.organicconsumers.org./news/hot-toxic-are-your-household-cleaning-supplies.

2021. Product Reviews.
https://www.Anthropologie.com.

2020. "Hand Sanitizer Can Kill Sperm but Don't Use It as Spermicide."
https://www.healthline.com/health.healthy-sex/does-hand-sanitizer-kill-sperm.

2020. "How Can You Prevent Harm From Cleaning and Household Products?"
https://www.lung.org/clean-air/at-home/indoor-air-pollutants/cleaning-supplies-household-chem.

2020. "Butylene Glycol."
https://www.thedermrevies.com/butylene-glycol.

2020. "Cleaning Supplies and Household Chemicals."
https://www.lung.org/clean-air/at-home/indoor-air-pollutants/cleaning-supplies-household-chem.

2019. "The Dangers Of Chemical Residue Left By Cleaning Products."
https://www.geneontechnologies.com/blog/the-dangers-of-chemical-residue-left-behind-by-cleaning-products.

2019. "Health Risks for Cleaners and Janitors."
https://www.geneontechnologies.com/blog/health-risks-for-cleaners-and-janitors.

2017. "Cleaning Chemicals: Know the Risks."
https://www.safetyandhealthmagazine.com/articles/16383-cleaning-chemicals-know-the-risks.

2009. "The List of 18 Toxic Cleaning Chemicals in Everyday Products." https://www.bigbluewaves.net/avoid-toxic-cleaning-chemicals.

Fukushima, Kurumi. (2020, July 28) "5 Hidden Dangers of Hand Sanitizers." https://www.thestreet.com/markets.

Hendon, Jeremy. 2020. "Is Your Hand Sanitizer Making You Infertile?" https://paleoflourish.com/hand-sanitizer-making-you-infertile/.

"The Hidden Dangers of Commercial Cleaning Residue." http://www.nationalpurity.com/the-hidden-dangers-of-commercial-cleaning-residue/.

Korab, Alek. 2020. "9 Side Effects of Using Hand Sanitizer, According to Doctors." https://www.eatthis.com/side-effects-hand-sanitizer-doctors/.

"Protecting Porkers Who Use Cleaning Chemicals; OSHA NIOSH Infosheet." https://www.osha.gov/sites/default/files/publications/OSHA3512.pdf.

MacPherson, Lynn. 2018. "Allergic Reaction to Hand Sanitizers." https://healthfully.com/allergic-reaction-to-hand-sanitizers.

McInnis, Kaitlyn. 2020. "The Scary Effect Using Too Much Sanitizer Can Have on Your Health." https://www.theladders.com/career-advice/the-scary-effect-using-too-much-sanitizer-can-have-on-your-health.

Settembre, Jeanette. 2020. "Hand Sanitizer Poisoning During Coronavirus Surges, Calls To Poison Control Up 70%." https://www.foxnews.com/health/hand-sanitizer-poisoning-coronavirus.

Shriver, Lauren. 2016. "Defining Green Cleaning and Why It's Important." https://www.cleanlink.com/news/article/Defining-Green-Cleaning-And-Why-It8217s-Important--20191.

The Memory Is the First To Go

Agrebi, Said, and Anis Larbi. *Artificial Intelligence in Precision Health*. Academic Press, 2020.

Davey, Basiro. *Immunology A Foundation Text*. New Jersey: Prentice Hall, 1990.

Fukushima, Kurumi. (2020, July 28) "5 Hidden Dangers of Hand Sanitizers." https://www.thestreet.com/markets.

Korab, Alek. 2020. "9 Side Effects of Using Hand Sanitizer, According to Doctors." https://www.eatthis.com/side-effects-hand-sanitizer-doctors/.

Henriques-Normark, Birgitta, and Staffan Normark. 2014. "Bacterial Vaccines and Antibiotic Resistance." *Upsala Journal of Medical Sciences* 119, no. 2: 205–8. doi:10.3109/03009734.2014.903324

Immunological Memory: Biology for Majors II. https://courses.lumenlearning.com/wm-

biology2/chapter/immunological-memory/.
Accessed 2021, April 8.

Shahi, Surkriti. 2019. "Global Handwashing Day
2019: 5 Side Effects of Hand Sanitizers You
Didn't Know About."
https://www.thehealthsite.com/diseases-
conditions/global-handwashng-day-1029.

An Educated Guess

Mayo Clinic. 2020. "Asthma."
https://www.mayoclinic.org/diseases-
conditions/asthma/symptoms-causes/syc-
20369653.

Bloomfield, SF, et al. 2006. "Too Clean, or Not Too
Clean: The Hygiene Hypothesis and Home
Hygiene." *Clinical and Experimental Allergy* 36,
no. 4: 402–425.

Craig, Christine Wilmsen. 2013. "Can You Develop
Allergies by Being Too Clean?"
https://www.aacos.com/blog/can-you-
develp-allergies-by-being-too-clean/.

Korab, Alek. 2020. "9 Side Effects of Using Hand
Sanitizer, According to Doctors."
https://www.eatthis.com/side-effects-hand-
sanitizer-doctors/.

London School of Hygiene & Tropical Medicine
(LSHTM). "Increase in allergies is not from
being too clean, just losing touch with 'old
friends." *ScienceDaily* (October 2012).
https://www.sciencedaily.com/releases/2012
/10/121003082734.

CDC. "Most Recent National Asthma Data."
https://www.cdc.gov/asthma/most-recent-national-asthma-data.

Richtel, Matt. 2019. "Your Environment Is Cleaner. Your Immune System Has Never Been So Unprepared."
https://www.nytimes.com/2019/03/12/health/immune-system-allergies.html.

Shahi, Surkriti. 2019. "Global Handwashing Day 2019: 5 Side Effects of Hand Sanitizers You Didn't Know About."
https://www.thehealthsite.com/diseases-conditions/global-handwashng-day-1029.

Stromberg, Joseph. 2015. "The Hygiene Hypothesis: How Being Too Clean Might Be Making Us Sick."
https://www.vox.com/2014/6/25/5837892/is-being-too-clean-making-us-sick.

Vann, Madeline. 2013. "Is Cleanliness Among the Causes of Allergies?"
https://www.everydayhealth.com/allergies/cleaning-and-allergies.aspx.

Yeomans, Tim. 2018. "Does Being Too Clean Cause Allergies?"
https://www.allergystandards.com/news_events/hygiene-hyypothesis/.

Super What??? Superbugs!!!

https://www.CDC.gov

Fukushima, Kurumi. 2020. "5 Hidden Dangers of
     Hand Sanitizers."
     https://www.thestreet.com/markets.
Mayo Clinic. "MRSA Infection."
     https://www.mayoclinic.org/diseases-
     conditions/mrsa/symptoms-causes/syc-
     20375336.
Neild, David. 2018. "Superbugs Are Growing More
     Resistant to Hand Sanitizer, Scientists Warn."
     https://sciencealert.com/superbugs-
     becoming-more-reisiant-to-hand-sanitizer.
Shahi, Surkriti. 2019. "Global Handwashing Day
     2019: 5 Side Effects of Hand Sanitizers You
     Didn't Know About."
     https://www.thehealthsite.com/diseases-
     conditions/global-handwashng-day-1029.
Stanborough, Rebecca Joy. 2020. "All about
     Superbugs and How To Protect Yourself
     from Them."
     https://www.healthline.com/health/superbug
     .

Out with the New, In with the Old

FARE. 2021. "Cleaning Methods."
     https://www.foodallergy.org/resources/clean
     ing-methods.
Gershman, Jennifer. 2017. "3 Things You Should
     Know about Ingestion of Alcohol-Based
     Hand Sanitizer."
     https://www.pharmacytimes.com/view/3-

things-you-should-know-about-ingestion-of-
alcohol-based-hand-sanitizer.

Getting the Last Word
Duerr, Charlie. 2020. "The CDC Says You Must
Keep Hand Sanitizer Away From Kids Under
This Age." https://bestlifeonline.com/hand-
sanitizer-kids-cdc/.
Fukushima, Kurumi. 2020. "5 Hidden Dangers of
Hand Sanitizers."
https://www.thestreet.com/markets.

Handwashing Day
CDC. 2019. "Global Handwashing Day 2019: Clean
Hands for All."
https://www.unwater.org/global-
handwashing-day-2019.
CDC. 2019. "Global Handwashing Day."
https://www.cdc.gov/handwashing/global-
handwashing-day.html.
Shahi, Surkriti. 2019. "Global Handwashing Day
2019: 5 Side Effects of Hand Sanitizers You
Didn't Know About."
https://www.thehealthsite.com/diseases-
conditions/global-handwashng-day-1029.

9 781737 532217